Guidebook

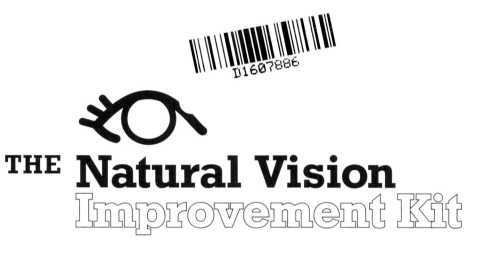

THE **Natural Vision** Improvement Kit

Meir Schneider, Ph.D., LMT

SOUNDS TRUE · BOULDER COLORADO

Sounds True, Inc. Boulder CO 80306
©2004 Meir Schneider

ISBN 1-59179-256-8

For a free catalog of wisdom teachings for the inner life, please contact
Sounds True
PO Box 8010
Boulder CO 80306-8010
800-333-9185
www.soundstrue.com

Meir Schneider, PhD, LMT is available for private sessions, or to teach vision
classes in your town or place of business. Please contact www.self-healing.org
or 415-665-9574.

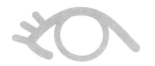

Table of Contents

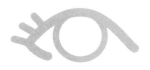

Introduction

While most of us know that we can improve our health and live longer by eating better, getting regular exercise, reducing stress, and practicing relaxation techniques, when it comes to our eyes we have a kind of learned helplessness. Very few of us believe there is anything we can do to make our eyes healthier, or to improve our eyesight. It is true that statistics show that most people who see poorly will never improve their eyesight, and that their vision will continue to deteriorate, but these statistics might look very different if we were taught how to take care of our eyes—or, even more importantly, if we understood that we have the power to improve our eyesight.

Western medical training puts great emphasis on the treatment of physical symptoms. If you see poorly, you are prescribed glasses that will correct your vision. If you have cataracts, doctors will remove the lens. If your have ocular hypertension or glaucoma, there are surgical procedures that will relieve pressure to your optic nerve.

Symptomatic solutions—lasik surgery, glasses, contact lenses, and other medical procedures that are performed to improve errors of refraction—do help you see better in the short term, but, ultimately, they only make your eyes weaker. Meanwhile, these remedies perpetuate the myth of helplessness that keeps you from strengthening your vision through natural vison self-care—an approach that has not only been effective for many thousands of people, but is far preferable in terms of both visual function and self-empowerment.

There is no question in my mind, after 30 years of working with all kinds of vision problems, that helping your eyesight is not simply an issue of getting rid of your glasses, but of dealing with your total being: your mental, emotional, and physical state in its entirety. This is why, when we begin working to improve our eyes, we need to approach this work from every possible angle. It is also why, in the process of doing so, you will discover things about yourself that you may never have suspected.

The Natural Vision Improvement approach is a kind of *yoga* for your eyes—a natural way of improving your eye health without the use of drugs, surgery, or devices that can act as crutches for poor vision. Using yoga for your eyes means learning to unite with your eyes by being present with them, exactly the way they are. When we unite with our eyes, we set aside our preconceptions and become curious about their true experience. We begin to pay attention to them, noticing when they are tired or irritated. As we would with any good friend, we attend to their needs: resting them when they have been working hard, and gently exercising them when they become weak or damaged.

In every situation, there is a better way to use your eyes. Sitting at your computer, standing in line at the bank, stalled in traffic—the exercises included in *The Natural Vision Improvement Kit* will teach you how to take advantage of this type of situation to work on your eyes. This program will also address many common eye problems, including the tension that leads to repetitive eyestrain related to computer use. This kit consists of this guidebook, 13 practice cards, and two guided exercise CDs. This guidebook is designed to give you an in-depth understanding of your vision, eye tension, and the techniques that can help you improve poor vision. The practice cards are numbered in the order they appear on the exercise CDs, and they can be used as a reference for the guided exercises. The first CD in the program is designed for anyone who uses computers, whether vision improvement is needed or not. The second CD is an introduction to the Natural Vision Improvement techniques that can help improve poor vision. Although some exercises are repeated on both CDs, each guided practice is tailored specifically for computer eyestrain relief or natural vision improvement. This program will also give you the tools you need to become more aware of your eyes and your power to heal them. If you practice these techniques with diligence, you will find yourself with healthier eyes and better vision, regardless of the present state of your eyes.

Ideally, you should devote at least an hour each day to the structured exercise program in *The Natural Vision Improvement Kit.* However, I believe you will find that even spending a few minutes daily with some of these exercises will yield measurable results, in the form of diminished eyestrain, clearer vision, and a greater ability to shift your focus without loss of clarity.

It has been my experience that, when people do these vision improvement exercises correctly—and devote to them the time they deserve—mild vision problems improve rapidly, and poor vision improves noticeably over a longer period. It is common to see improvements in even the first session, but it takes longer to stabilize these gains. The brief flashes of better vision are a hallmark of impending change.

True eye health is not a matter of abandoning your computer or abandoning your present lifestyle. By all means, continue to do whatever is necessary to perform your job, but also realize that, in order to function at your best, it is important to incorporate these eye exercises into your daily routine. You do not have to cut down on your reading, but you should learn to incorporate these techniques and practices into your daily life if you want to fully enjoy and engage with your lifestyle. In fact, the most important change does not have to do with your activities at all—the most important aspect of this program is a new understanding of the relationship you have with your eyes and your brain. By beginning this program, you have already taken a step in which the benefits will expand, beyond even improving your eyesight and eye health, into a new relationship to your life—a relationship based on awareness, acceptance, and true harmony.

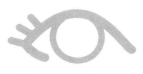

Chapter One
Dr. William H. Bates— Ophthalmologic Visionary

Before we begin this work, let us explore how the work of Natural Vision Improvement came about. I was born with cataracts and other serious vision problems. By the time I was seven years of age, I had undergone five operations to remove the cataracts. While the surgeries removed most of the cataracts, they shattered my lenses and created dense scar tissue. The doctors pronounced my condition hopeless, and I was certified as legally blind. I could see only light, shadow, and indistinct shapes, and I performed all of my schoolwork and reading in Braille. At the age of seventeen, I learned the Bates Method of eye exercises and practiced them with a diligence that probably no one had ever applied to them before, spending up to 13 hours a day practicing. My vision dramatically improved and today, I am licensed to drive a car without the help of glasses or contact lenses.

The exercises you will learn in *The Natural Vision Improvement Kit* are inspired by the Bates Method, with refinements and additions developed during three decades of reversing my own blindness and helping others work with their visual problems. These methods have been proven effective in relieving all refractive conditions (any structural problem affecting the trajectory of light within the eye), and in correcting squints and lazy eyes, and similar problems. They do not necessarily address eye diseases, but they do help you nurture healthier eyes that are more resistant to disease and better able to heal themselves from any reversible condition.

You may have heard of the Bates Method: a series of exercises designed to strengthen eyesight without the use of glasses. Its creator is Dr. William H. Bates, who was born in 1860 and graduated from Cornell University's College of Physicians and Surgeons at the age of thirty-five. Three years later, he was serving his internship at Columbia Hospital in New York as an ear, nose, throat, and eye doctor (in those days, these specialties were combined). Dr. Bates was working as a teaching assistant, but was dismissed after repeatedly encouraging fellow doctors to go without the glasses prescribed for them by the chief ophthalmologist at the hospital eye clinic.

Dr. Bates used an instrument called the *retinoscope,* with which he could observe minute changes in the surface curvature of the eye, and thereby determine the nature and degree of a patient's vision problems. Over many years, he observed the eyes of hundreds of patients in every kind of activity, emotional state, and physical condition. He noted how their eyes changed when they were doing work they enjoyed, or when they were doing work they disliked. He also noted the differences in their eyes when they were fatigued, anxious, or confused, and when they were focused, excited, stimulated, or relaxed.

You have probably noticed that your vision is better at some times and worse at others. Among the discoveries Dr. Bates made was that visual clarity changes—in the same person—from good to bad and back again, depending on that person's physical and emotional state. He concluded that vision is not a static condition, but one that changes constantly.

His research shows how vision defects can be created and/or worsened by the stress of everyday situations. He also proved that these problems can be corrected by conscious and correct visual behavior.

Dr. Bates died in 1931, having spent his life researching and developing a method to relieve the unnecessary suffering of people afflicted with eye disorders. His compassion and concern for his patients was legendary. Upon seeing an infant fitted with tiny glasses, Dr. Bates remarked, "It is enough to make the angels weep."

Chapter Two

The Body-Mind Connection

What Is Vision?

To improve your vision, you first need to change the way you think about seeing, as well as the way you go about seeing. Our dependence on sight is enormous, especially in people who see well. When these people lose their good vision, it can be very traumatic, changing their entire self-concept. In reality, such people have great resources to help them restore their vision, and you will find these resources explained and demonstrated in the exercises included in *The Natural Vision Improvement Kit.*

The eye is one of the most used muscles in our bodies, but it is not simply a mechanical tool. Like every other part of the body, it is profoundly affected by your state of mind. In fact, vision is the sum total of sensation, perception, and conception. Mechanically speaking, your retina has about 126 million light-sensing photoreceptor cells that produce nearly one billion images every minute. Your brain cannot possibly assimilate all of those images to create a picture, so it selects which ones to concentrate on—basically determining how much of a picture you will see.

The British writer Aldous Huxley was a successful student and enthusiastic admirer of Dr. Bates' method. After using his exercises to recover from a condition of near-blindness, Huxley wrote a book called *The Art of Seeing,* in which he described seeing as a three-step process involving the eyes, the brain, and the mind. He explained that seeing consists of:

Sensing: The light-sensitive cells of the eyes receive information about their environment via light rays—approximately one billion bits of visual data during any given second.

Selecting: The mind cannot deal with all of the visual data being conveyed to the eyes, so it directs the eyes to pay attention only to certain data.

Perceiving: The selected visual data are recognized and interpreted by the mind.

Visual improvement requires that we recognize vision as a complex interaction between the eyes and the mind. We also need to learn how to make the mind work for us, rather than against us.

One of the biggest obstacles we need to overcome is the belief that the eyes can never improve. This belief can keep us from recognizing or accepting improvement when it does occur, or convince us that in certain situations we simply will not be able to see, and therefore should not try.

Sometimes our vision may worsen when we expect it to—in situations where we feel our eyes are being challenged. Dr. Bates described a situation in which he had two of his patients—one with excellent vision and the other with poor vision—look at a blank wall. During this experiment, he monitored changes in the surface curvature of their eyes with his retinoscope. As long as both patients looked at the blank wall, their eyes remained the same. As soon as he placed an eye chart on the wall, the eyes of the person with poor vision changed radically, with all of the surrounding muscles contracting sharply. The eyes of the person with good vision showed only a slight, barely noticeable change. The first one had immediately and unconsciously brought his habits of straining into his effort to see the chart.

Visual habits and patterns of use are among the hardest to change; in fact, we are more attached to the way we see than to almost anything else we do. Perhaps this is because our memory consists mostly of visual information. Once we have seen something in a certain way, we remember it that way and continue to see it as we remember it.

Memory and imagination are the mind's most valuable tools for improving vision. Anything we have ever seen clearly can be used to stimulate clearer vision. We all know that it is easier to see things that are known and familiar. For example, an unfamiliar word, though it is made up of the same letters, will initially be harder to decipher than a familiar one. We use visualization exercises to take advantage of the mind's tendency to associate clear vision with that which is known and familiar. We can also use visualization or imagination to create optimal conditions. Imagining total blackness, for example, can cause the optic nerve to react as though it were, in fact, seeing total blackness—that is, to stop working and rest.

Your Eyes and Your Brain

Theories that blame eye structure for the origin of our visual problems are very limited, in that they do not recognize the profound body-mind dynamics that cause the structural changes to begin with. Conventional ophthalmology holds that structure creates function; this is why poor vision is typically treated with instruments or surgeries designed to change the structure of the eye. But the truth is that all vision begins with thought. Your thoughts dictate how your eyes function, and the way your eyes function changes their structure. If you learn to function differently with your mind, you may also change the structure of your eye.

The most important visual organ is the brain. The mind, like any other powerful force of nature, can either help or harm. It can keep us from believing that our vision can improve, or it can supply us with everything we need to improve it. The eyes and the brain even share the same kinds of tissue. Our sensitive eyes respond to the minutest chemical changes in the brain—including those caused by emotional states and mental events.

The extent of your brain's control over visual function is evident in the way it makes sense of impressions that your eyes alone cannot interpret. For example: physics teaches that, although you perceive objects as right side up, your lens and retina are seeing them upside down. Your eyes have no mechanical function that translates the upside-down images into the perspective you normally see. It is your brain that needs to put everything right side up, to create order in the world. A startling experiment illuminates this point quite vividly.

A group of pilots was given glasses that made everything appear upside down. Within a couple of days, their brains righted their vision and they saw everything right side up again, even through their glasses. Two weeks later, the glasses were taken away. Everything turned upside down. With time, they all saw things right side up again without the glasses.

Your Eyes and Your Emotions

Vision is also very much a result of your emotional state. Almost every client I have worked with has experienced strong emotions—and sometimes powerful emotional insights—while working to improve their vision. Conversely, strong negative emotions nearly always worsen vision temporarily. This is true even for people with good eyesight. If the emotional stress continues, damage to the eyes can become permanent.

I have learned that visual deterioration is often due to an unwillingness to observe the world closely. When we are under emotional stress, the last thing we want to do is look at the details of our situation. It is less painful, at times like this, to partially "blind" ourselves to the reality of our experience. Our vision becomes fuzzy in an attempt to protect us emotionally. Our eyes lose their ability to "shift" from one detail to another, resulting in a frozen stare that stresses our eyes tremendously. Unfortunately, our typical reaction to this situation is to force our eyes to perform as usual. We acquire glasses, or get a stronger prescription.

If you strained your back by using it to lift heavy objects, you would not think of just getting a back brace and continuing to use your spine in the same way. Yet this is precisely how we treat our eyes. It would be much better for your long-term visual health if you simply acknowledged your need to see less clearly for a while. This is a time to rest and support your eyes, your body, and your mind. In a world dedicated to functionality, this might be difficult to do—yet to ignore physical and emotional distress signals is to risk permanent damage to your ability to function. If you nurture your eyesight through the hard times, it will return to its previous capacity when things start (literally) looking up again.

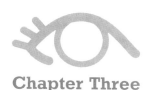

Chapter Three

The Causes of Poor Vision

Vision problems usually manifest as a lack of clarity in either near or distant vision. The physical act of seeing things close up is different from that of seeing things in the distance. Consider, for example, how a camera works. When light rays from the object you are photographing reach the camera's lens, they need to converge so that they are focused on the film behind the lens. To focus, you change the distance between the lens and the film until it is just right—otherwise the light rays will not focus exactly on the film, and the image will be blurred.

In the same way, your eye needs to converge light rays from the object you are looking at and focus them behind the lens. Instead of film, these light rays need to focus on your *retina,* which is a network of nerve cells in the rear of the eye itself that translates the light rays into neural information. These data are sent through the optic nerve to the brain. Whereas a camera has the ability to change the distance between the lens and the film, the eye changes the shape of the lens instead. When the thin *ciliary muscles* that surround the lens and hold it in place are relaxed, the lens is relatively flat and allows for distant vision. When the object you are looking at is closer than 20 feet away, those muscles contract, and the lens assumes a more spherical shape. This process is called accommodation (*see Figure A*).

Shape of the Eye

Another factor thought to determine how a person sees is the shape of the eyeball. Irregularly shaped eyeballs are considered the cause of two common vision problems: *myopia* and *hyperopia.* Myopia (nearsightedness) means the inability to see distant objects clearly, caused by an eyeball that is too long from front to back. This shape makes it impos-

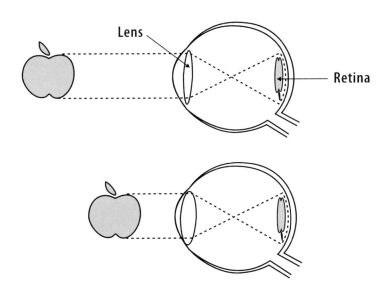

FIGURE A How an eye works: when the object is close, the lens changes shape, becoming more spherical.

sible for the lens to focus the light rays from distant objects onto the retina (*see Figure B*), though it can focus the rays from close objects. *Hyperopia*—or *hypermetropia* (farsightedness)—refers to the inability to see close objects clearly. Here, the eyeball is too short from front to back. Light rays from a distance focus correctly, but the lens is unable to bring the rays together before they reach the retina. If they were capable of passing through it, the rays would probably focus behind the retina (*see Figure C*).

These descriptions explain the mechanical conditions underlying poor vision, but what causes these physical changes to occur? The answer is *eye tension*. The eyes are as susceptible to tension and stress as any other part of the body, and are subjected to at least as much of it.

Eye Tension

Many people think tension is a trivial matter. Tension is often considered a temporary condition that will not do damage to the muscles and nerves that it taxes.

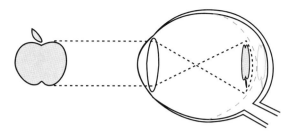

FIGURE B Myopia is caused by an eyeball that is too long from front to back. The lens cannot focus distant objects onto the retina, creating a blurry image.

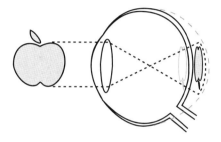

FIGURE C Hyperopia is caused by an eyeball that is too short from front to back. The lens focuses close objects beyond the retina, creating a blurry image.

Truthfully, tension is one of the worst afflictions from which you can suffer. Because its effect is underestimated and often goes unnoticed, tension can often be the root cause of poor vision.

The two components of visual stress—*tasks with high-level cognitive demand* and *prolonged, unrelieved near-focusing*—often coincide with our modern ways of living.

Many of our actions and reactions—as well as much of our memory—are guided by mental pictures, including conscious and subconscious images of events that shaped our emotional makeup. Our eyes are stressed even when we perceive these images only "in the mind's eye." All of these events take place in the brain, of which the eye is an integral part. Because of all this, and also because we use them for just about everything we do, our eyes respond strongly to our thoughts and emotions. Many people engage in a daily routine that requires a high level of cognitive thinking. They have learned to carry a great many responsibilities by multi-tasking throughout the day. This can create a high-level of stress on both the mind and body.

The effects of near focusing and computer use on the eyes

The advent of computers has compounded this problem. A typical person might spend 8 to 10 hours at work in front of their computer, only to go home and surf the internet for another 2 to 3 hours. There is little or no break from looking at the near field view of the computer. It is estimated that there are over 105 million people who use computers daily in this country. Ophthalmologists estimate that over 70 million of those people suffer from a condition called *repetitive eyestrain* (RSI), which is an inflammation of the tissue and nerves surrounding the eyes. In general, this condition is caused by chronic eye tension. In addition, many of these people suffer from a visual/postural repetitive strain condition called *Computer Vision Syndrome* (CVS). Symptoms include eyestrain, general fatigue, neck and shoulder pain, dry eyes, and difficulties in focusing.

When the eyes are strained through prolonged computer use, an unnecessary burden is put on them. The cells in the eye mechanism become weak and deteriorate from the strain because they are not given periodic breaks in order to recover. When this eye tension becomes chronic, it leads to eye problems, and sometimes to eye pathologies like glaucoma or cataracts.

The computer screen is itself a visual stressor. Since the eye can never determine the focal length of computer pixels, it is plunged into a visual limbo in which the muscles surrounding the lens (the ciliary muscles) continually quiver with unavailing effort. The visual stress of CVS tends to bring on myopia or make it worse. While it is possible to harm your eyes by using the computer in an unconscious way, it is also important to realize that, by changing your habits now, you can prevent many of problems that can occur.

When you strain your eyes in front of a computer, a few things can go wrong:

Your peripheral view is limited. When you are looking at a computer screen, your focused field of vision includes only the screen and the words on that screen. When the two peripheries (left and right) are not being used, the central vision has too heavy of a burden. A concentrated amount of tension develops on the central retina that, over time, causes the central retina to become weak and withered. This can also cause one eye to work harder than the other and create an imbalanced use of the two eyes. The healthiest use of the eyes is one that uses both eyes, the periphery of both eyes, and the central retina of both eyes in a balanced manner.

You stop blinking. When focusing in the near field of the computer screen, you strain your eyes to the extent that you stop blinking at a normal rate. It has been shown that people who use the computer daily blink only seven times per minute, while people who do not use a computer daily (or not at all) blink 22 times per minute. Blinking massages and lubricates the eyes and creates a more relaxed state for mind and body.

Your eye muscles are continually contracted. When looking at a computer screen, you are focusing in the near field of your vision. To see things that are near, the ciliary muscles that surround the pupils contract and the lens becomes convex (*see Figure D*). In a healthy person, looking in the near field of vision for 1 to 3 hours in a day is a great way to strengthen the ciliary muscles. However, when using a computer, you are often looking at the screen for 8 to 12 hours a day. This prolonged near-field looking causes a great deal of stress in the ciliary muscles. Because of the contraction that occurs all day long, when you finally look in the far field of vision, the muscles are unable to relax and allow the lens to be flat. This is one of the main

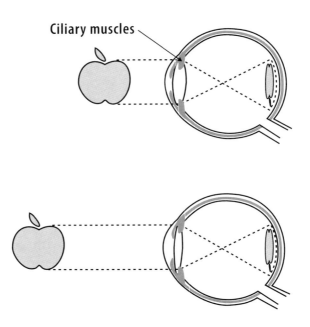

FIGURE D How the ciliary muscles work: When the eye looks in the near field of vision, the ciliary muscles contract to make the lens convex. When the eye looks in the far field of vision, the ciliary muscles relax to make the lens flatten.

reasons why so many people need to wear glasses, but, in a long-term sense, wearing corrective lens is not the proper solution to this type of eyestrain.

Your pupils lose their flexibility. When you look at the computer all day long, there is no differentiation in the shades of light that you see, and your eyes are exposed to a constant light that does not change. Therefore, the pupil does not get the experience of expanding and contracting to different shades of light as the day passes, and the pupil becomes stiff as a result. The pupils are muscles, and when they are not given the full range of mobility from expansion to contraction, eventually they become inflexible and slow to react to light stimuli. From ancient times until 200 years ago, humans who spent time outdoors were exposed to many dynamic shades of light, which infrequently occurs for today's modern person. Even if you have a window in your workspace, it is likely that your mind drives you to look at what is most interesting—the content of your computer screen.

Poor Circulation

Another consideration in causes of poor vision is poor circulation. As we get older, we become more engrained in our habits of stress and tightness, not only in the eyes, but in the body. Muscle tightness in the areas of the head, neck, and shoulders causes less blood to come into the eye cells. This can lead to *neo-vacuolization,* which occurs when additional blood vessels form in the retina because not enough blood is flowing to the eyes. The unfortunate consequence is that those vessels are imperfect and leak, which can cause blindness unless proper medical treatment is given. Poor circulation should not be ignored, as it can perpetuate eye tension and poor vision.

Stress and Eye Health

Stress and poor vision are interconnected. When the body and mind are stressed, the body, face, and eyes reflect that stress with muscle tension. This tension can lead to poor eyesight. Poor eyesight can then lead to self-consciousness and further emotional stress. To break this cycle of poor eyesight creating tension and tension creating worsening eyesight, we have to shift our consciousness and change our habits.

People with bad vision often believe that they were born to see poorly, and that nothing they can do will cause their vision to be better or worse. But our living habits—which begin at an early age and continue into adulthood—have a direct impact on our eye health. It has been shown that illiterate societies have much better eyesight than those who are more literate. In literate Hong Kong, 62% of children need glasses, whereas in rural Tibet, where illiteracy is common, only 3% have poor vision.

Because of eyestrain, most people wear glasses sooner or later. We do not go outdoors enough, and too many indoor hours are spent at the computer. Many people with perfect vision begin to have poor vision subsequent to eyestrain and, once they begin to wear glasses, their vision becomes even worse.

The atmosphere of stress in the workplace can also contribute to eye tension, and many people are not even aware of this tension. The subliminal effects of this tension can cause the deterioration of vision to escalate.

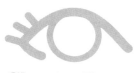

Chapter Four
The Fundamentals
of Natural Vision Improvement

Our primitive ancestors used all their senses—including their vision—fully. They looked into the distance; they noticed the slightest movement at the far periphery of their vision. Their eyes shifted constantly from detail to detail, from close up to far away. They could find their way both in the dark and in the full light of day.

Sadly, our reality today is not nearly so fluid. Life hardens our bodies. When we work hard, we tense our posture and contract. When we read or work at the computer, the rest of the room is of no interest to us. We spend most of our days staring at work just a few inches from our noses. Daylight blinds us when we step outdoors after working indoors all day; we find ourselves straining to see in the dark.

These bad visual habits lead to a "frozen" look: a gaze that basically discounts much of the visual field. We do not use the larger portion of the visual capacity and acuity naturally available to us—and in time, the brain reinforces this behavior and fixates the eye around it. In this way, it creates a predictable reality in which we expect to see only certain things and only in certain ways. It imposes its visual memory to recreate our visual experiences in the moment.

In this program, you will learn how to develop what I call *soft eyes:* eyes that are truly open to whatever there is to see. The concept of soft eyes was developed by martial arts practitioners to describe the kind of vision necessary in order to be aware of three opponents coming at you from different directions. With a frozen gaze, you would only be able to focus on one at a time, which would lead very quickly to your defeat.

By contrast, soft eyes have great presence. They take in the whole room, the whole landscape, without straining for any particular visual impression. Looking with soft eyes is similar to taking a walk for the pure pleasure of moving your body, without scheming over the calories you are burning or the muscles you are toning. Soft eyes absorb the world, rather than trying to capture it; your eyes rest while you look, rather than strain. With soft eyes, the process of looking is as important as the content of what is seen. Obviously, this is a much more relaxed approach to living than the one most of us are used to.

The Guidelines for Natural Vision Improvement

You should work with the following guidelines whenever you do the exercises and throughout the day. Practice these suggestions, and you will find that your eyes are surprisingly responsive to your nurturing attention.

Never, under any circumstances, strain to see anything. It is impossible to force better vision—in fact, trying to do so will reverse all of the benefits you derive from these exercises. Instead, notice what you do see, and use that information to enhance your exercises.

Let your vision be what it is. If it is blurred, do not try to make it clear. Simply work with what you have and notice what mental, physical, and emotional conditions contribute to changes in your eyesight. (You do not have to change these conditions, by the way; just being aware of them will start a natural process of change.)

Do not force yourself to do any exercise that feels uncomfortable to you. Discuss any qualms you may have with your ophthalmologist, and use your own judgment and intuition to personalize the program for your unique needs.

Goals are a setup for disappointment and frustration. Imposing a schedule on your visual improvement is counterproductive. Discover your own pace and respect it; this is truly the fastest way to improve your eyesight.

Remember that your eyes are not isolated from the rest of your body. If your back hurts, or your neck is tense, or you do not eat well, your eyes will respond to these stresses by losing function. Make the exercises in this program a part of an overall program for nurturing your body, mind, and spirit.

The Basic Principles of Natural Vision Improvement

There are many ways you can work on your eyes. Some techniques concentrate specifically on a particular aspect of visual function, others focus on the health of your eyes, and still others look at your overall well-being. Ideally, your daily workout will touch on all these elements—but in order to understand the program more clearly, we can group all the exercises into five basic categories:

- Relaxation
- Adjusting to varying intensity of light
- Balancing your eyes
- Flexibility of the lens
- Working the eyes and the body together

Relaxation

The eye is one of the hardest-working organs in the body, and people who use their eyes a lot become fatigued more rapidly than others. This partially explains why a typist can be as exhausted as a lumberjack at the end of a workday.

We use our eyes every minute we are awake—typically, about 17 hours daily. Imagine how your muscles would feel if you used them nonstop, every waking moment. If you work at a job that requires constant and strenuous use of your eyes—as many of us do—consider how your body would feel if you forced it to walk all day, every day, under the weight of a heavy burden. Yet, this is exactly the kind of pressure we put on our eyes.

You might feel that you relax your eyes for many hours each day, while you sleep. The fact is that during much of our sleep time, our eyes are not resting enough. During dreams, the optic nerve is stimulated, and the eyes are in motion under our closed eyelids. It has been clearly established that all humans spend several hours a night in this state. In addition, many people do not relax during sleep, but maintain their tensions—particularly in the upper body and face.

Ideally, you should be able to improve your vision through both use and rest. Everything you do with your eyes should be good for them. One of the most important things you can do for them is simply to counteract the abuse to which they are typically subjected. The most effective way to accomplish this is through relaxation.

Your eyes are an integral part of your body. It is unrealistic to think you can relax them when the rest of your body is tense. This is why *The Natural Vision Improvement Kit* begins with looking far at a distance, self-massage, and other relaxation techniques.

Adjusting to varying intensity of light
Light is the vehicle that brings all visual information to your eyes. People who spend much of their time working outdoors under bright, natural light tend to have better eyesight than those of us who live mostly indoors, because their eyes are accustomed to—and comfortable with—strong light. They can accept and use the light fully. The more time we spend under dim, inadequate, artificial lighting, the less our eyes are equipped to deal with light in general. Normal sunlight can feel like a spotlight shone into your face. This is partly because spending most of your time indoors forces your pupils to chronically dilate, opening as wide as possible in order to take in all available light. The muscles around your eyes will tend to tighten, squinting to shut out the painful glare. Many people are currently walking around with sunglasses or with a perpetual, unconscious squint shielding their eyes from "excess" light.

To some extent, squinting works temporarily. Its long-term effects, however, are very detrimental to vision. It causes the muscles around the eyes to constantly contract, which changes the shape of the eyeball. It also cuts out a large part of the peripheral visual field, forcing the eyes to stare fixedly, with effort, at a very small area. In this situation, sunglasses are about as helpful as a wheelchair to a person with weak leg muscles: they provide temporary relief, but ultimately serve only to further weaken the eyes' ability to cope with light.

Of course, I am not suggesting that you get rid of your sunglasses forever. You may still need them if you happen to be driving toward the setting sun. But if you regularly practice Natural Vision Improvement, you will need them less and less. Your eyes will accept much more light, much more comfortably. Your pupils will become more flexible, able to dilate and contract easily and quickly, making the transition from dark to light less painful. Your face will lose its squint, and your visual field will expand. You will no longer be blinded by the light of day.

Balancing your eyes

People with poor vision commonly do two things that lead to unbalanced use of the eyes: they allow one eye to dominate, and they use only their central vision while neglecting their peripheral vision. This behavior is, of course, completely unconscious—but it can be changed by conscious retraining.

Most of us tend to have a stronger, or *dominant,* eye. People with myopia know about this phenomenon, because their prescription is typically stronger for one eye than for the other. When one eye tends to dominate, the result is exactly the same as when we use only a few muscles to do the work of the entire body. The weaker, or *non-dominant,* eye is underused, and consequently weakens further, while the stronger eye works ceaselessly until it, too, begins to lose its strength.

Stimulating peripheral vision is intimately connected with balancing your stronger and weaker eye. When we look straight ahead with both eyes, it is easy to unconsciously let one eye do all the work. When we work with our periphery, however, we create a separate visual field for each eye, and so are much more apt to notice if one eye is not working.

Exercising your peripheral vision also helps to break the bad habits you may have established in overusing your central vision. The ancient Romans were entertained in amphitheaters, where their attention was attracted to objects at many points in a wide visual field. Today, our entertainment mostly requires us to look straight ahead: at television, a movie screen, or a stage. Contemporary optometry accepts 70% of our possible peripheral vision as within normal limits—in other words, most of us are missing about 30% of our available usage. Overuse of our central vision causes *ocular hypertension:* fluid comes into the eye faster than it can drain, slowly building up pressure on the optic nerve. Another name for this condition is *glaucoma.*

One more excellent reason to stimulate peripheral vision is that it tends to improve night vision because the same cells of the retina are involved.

Flexibility of the lens

The lens of the eye contracts and expands to see detail. When you look at something in the near field of your vision, your lens will contract in order to see it in greatest detail. Likewise, when you look at something far off in the distance, your lens will expand.

As we have already discussed, the modern person looks in their near field of vision for long periods of time throughout the day, which creates a contracted lens. This causes the lens itself to become less flexible when it expands to look at distant objects. When looking in the far field of vision, the lens becomes stiff and hard to mobilize into an expanded state. This inflexibility can be the cause of poor vision and even lead to cataracts later in life.

Working the eyes and body together

It is very important to work the eyes and body together. Why? To show the body that your eyes can really see. You will learn various exercises in this program that will feel difficult when you initially try them because you will do them without glasses or contacts and, in some cases, with your non-dominant eye. It is important to approach these exercises with an attitude of non-judgment and light-heartedness. The goal in all of these exercises is to demonstrate to the body that even without the crutch of glasses or contacts or even when the weaker eye is doing the work, that you can see and move the body in response to what you see. Only when the body understands that it can function with the sight that you already have, will your brain allow your sight to improve.

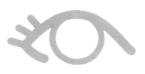

Chapter Five

A Final Word About Vision

The most important thing for you to know is that your vision is okay as it is. Whether you have so-called "perfect vision" or are legally blind, it is important to accept your present level of sight have compassion for yourself. Also, remember that your vision, like your body, has natural fluctuations of good and bad health. So always start where you are. The more you put pressure on yourself to see as well as someone else or see as well as you may with your glasses or contacts on, the more unconscious tension you are putting on yourself, which will negatively affect your vision-improvement efforts.

When you do the exercises that require the use of the eye charts, do not measure your eye health by measuring your vision with your glasses or contacts on, but rather, take them off and start off at a distance that feels most comfortable to you. Be patient with yourself and refrain from judgement. Improvement takes time and dedication.

Also, be aware of how your emotional and mental state affects your vision. Many people experience deteriorating vision during their college years, when there is a sense of confusion about what the future holds. Alternately, many people in their forties and fifties begin to experience farsightedness, or a difficulty seeing near. It is possible at this time in a person's life that they are reexamining the big picture, and are not so intensely focused on what is happening in the immediate future.

To a great extent, working on the eyes will trigger many emotional responses within the psyche, and I would like to recommend that, during your work in this program, you keep a journal and use it as a way of reflecting on your own individual experience of growth and discovery. You may be surprised at how the world may transform before you.

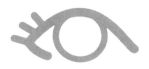

Chapter Six

Cautions and Contraindications: Please Read this Before Beginning Your Exercises

If you follow the Natural Vision Improvement program as set out in this kit, there is no downside. These practices produce no unhealthy side effects or added stress to other parts of your body-mind. There are, however, some cautions you must observe in order to protect your eyes while exercising. If you ignore the cautions listed below, you will miss the full benefits of the program. In some cases, you could actually cause real damage. Please take a moment to read this section each time you begin your exercise routine, at least for the first few days. As your eyes begin to feel comfortable with these new activities, your awareness will naturally keep you from employing counter-productive and dangerous practices.

Exercise tips
Please remove your glasses, sunglasses, or contact lenses while doing all of the following exercises. If you regularly alternate between glasses and contacts during your day, wear your glasses, so that you can take them off easily for the exercises. If you wear contacts, make sure you keep your contact solution and case nearby, so you can take your contacts out easily. However, if you find yourself entrenched in a busy work schedule that does not allow you to easily take your contacts out during your day, go ahead and do the exercises with your contacts in. It is better to do the exercises while wearing your contacts than not at all. The only exercise which should *never* be done with contacts in is sunning.

    Keep the cards close at hand so you can refer to them for tips on posture and technique.

Use a portable CD player and headphones for the outdoor portions of the guided practices until you become more familiar with the exercises and can do them on your own.

Remember to always breathe deeply and slowly while doing the exercises. The goal is to relax and relieve tension from the eyes and to increase the circulation to the eyes. Breathing will help facilitate this.

Pay attention to how your eyes feel as you practice. It is important to do the exercises mindfully, so that you can slowly develop a sense of what your eyes need at any given moment. These techniques are not mechanical exercises to be engaged in while your thoughts are elsewhere. These exercises are designed to work with your entire body-mind in such a way that they will create profound changes in your visual habits—in fact, they will change how you look at the world altogether.

If you wear glasses or contact lenses and are doing the exercises to improve your vision, do not expect to throw them away in the next few days. In time, you may find that you need a weaker prescription, or possibly no longer need your prescribed lenses at all. Still, using your glasses or contacts is preferable to squinting and straining in order to work or read. If your driver's license requires you to wear glasses while driving, continue to do so until you can pass the vision test at the Department of Motor Vehicles. Otherwise, experiment with using and not using your glasses or lenses as you proceed with the program. Let your guiding principle be how much you are able to keep your eyes relaxed in various situations. The more you learn to see adequately with relaxed eyes, the less you will need to use "corrective" lenses.

Any of the exercises in this program can be used separately for on-the-spot relief of eye tension or vision improvement. Use the guided audio sessions and/or practice cards to refer to until you can perform the exercise on your own.

Keep the cards handy at home and in your office so you will be reminded to do these exercises often.

In some exercises, you may be instructed to gather additional materials before you begin. Additional items you may need:

- A brightly colored ball or a tennis ball
- Masking tape
- A blanket and pillows
- A portable CD player and headphones for more mobility while doing the exercises

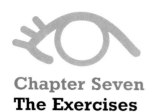

Chapter Seven

The Exercises

Exercise One: Looking Far at a Distance

The eyes are designed for a healthy balance of looking both in the near and far fields of vision, as when hunting and farming were a way of life. With the advent of computers, books, and other changes in our lifestyle, the average person now spends the majority of their day looking in the near field of their vision.

When you look in the near field of vision, the ciliary muscles around the lens contract to make the lens convex (*see Figure D, page 18*). Conversely, when you look away at something far at a distance, the ciliary muscles relax, and there is a flattening of the lens that requires no effort. It becomes a wonderful exercise for the total eyeball, because when you look far at a distance, the total eyeball itself becomes a bit shorter than when you are looking at your near field of vision. In this way, to look far at a distance, is the most natural and relaxing exercise that your eye can have. In addition, there is usually no mental activity involved when you are looking at a distance (such as when you are reading or working at a computer), so you can mentally relax as well, and simply enjoy whatever the eye sees.

Instructions while at the computer
Practicing looking at a distance when inside: If you are in a room with a window, with a soft gaze, locate four points on the horizon—like clouds or colors or features of the landscape. Let your eyes shift softly from one point to the next at your own pace, remembering to keep your gaze soft. If you are nearsighted and cannot see details at a distance, you may find yourself automatically straining to see the detail, or squinting to adjust to the light. Fight this urge and *do not squint*. Consciously relax your eyes and let your

eyes rest on whatever they see, whether the image is clear or blurry. Remember, the point of this exercise is to let your eyes relax and allow your lens to flatten. Breathe deeply. Enjoy what you see. Let this be a time of relaxation for your eyes and mind.

If you do not have a window, pick four points that are the farthest from where you are sitting in your room or office. Let your eyes shift from one point to the next, and let your gaze be soft. Remember to breathe deeply and enjoy the relaxation of looking far at a distance.

Instructions for outside

When outside: Keeping your gaze soft and remembering not to squint, pick four points on the horizon, and let your eyes shift softly from one point to the next at your own pace. You may need to face away from the sun to make sure you do not squint. Breathe deeply and slowly, allowing the fresh air to bring oxygen to your tense eyes. Relax your eyes, and let your eyes rest on whatever they see, whether the image is clear or blurry. Enjoy what you see. Let this be a time of relaxation for your eyes and mind.

Every minute or so, wave your hands to the side of your face as you continue to let your eyes softly rest on the horizon. This stimulates your peripheral vision. Begin to softly massage around your eye orbits—alternating between the right and left every few minutes—as you continue to look far at a distance. Let your fingertips softly massage the tension that has built up around your eyes. Begin at the bridge of your nose and massage underneath your eye orbits from the cheekbones to the temples. As you continue to breathe deeply and look at the horizon, pick four points that are a quarter of the distance closer to you, and begin to shift your gaze from one point to another while periodically massaging around the eye orbits and waving your hands to the side to stimulate your peripheral vision. You can continue to pick four points and decrease the distance you are gazing at, until 7 minutes have passed.

Variation: When you are outdoors looking at a distance, after about 3 to 4 minutes, take the small black piece of paper and some masking tape, and obstruct your dominant eye (*see page 52*). Keeping your gaze, look far at a distance.

MORE INFORMATION ABOUT this exercise, and a guided version of this practice are included as tracks 2 and 3 of CD 1, Learning to Relax the Ciliary Muscles, and Looking Far at a Distance While at the Computer

How often should I do this exercise?

When sitting in front of the computer: Try to do this exercise every 10 minutes for 15 to 30 seconds. Although this is the most frequent exercise you will do throughout your day, it takes less than a minute, and is a wonderful rest for your eyes. You can even use your computer to help set a reminder to do this. Many email and scheduling software programs have a setting that can play a chime or bell to remind you to take this much-needed break at scheduled times throughout the day.

When outside: When you are first learning the exercises of this program, it is important to be diligent in doing them. For the first 3 weeks after you begin, go outside three to four times a day and look for 7 minutes at a time. You can do this at the beginning of the day, during a lunch break, and before you go home, for example. Once you feel comfortable with this exercise, try the variation described above.

After the first 3 weeks of doing these exercises, you can reduce the frequency to once a day for 7 minutes at a time, again using the small piece of paper to stimulate and balance your eyes.

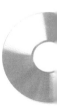

A GUIDED VERSION of this exercise is included as track 4 of CD 1, Looking Far at a Distance While Outside

Exercise Two: Facial Massage

Facial tension often stems from tension that begins in the eyes. When the muscles of the eye become tense—whether it is the pupilary muscles, the ciliary muscles, or the external muscles surrounding the eye—the muscles in the forehead, jaw, and neck become very tight, as well. It is as if the muscles of the face are trying to participate in the act of seeing by doing the contracting that the pupil should be doing. The brain then basically follows a habitual pattern that is familiar to itself, and makes a connection between the tension in the eyes and tension in the rest of the face and neck. So it is important to reintroduce the brain to the state of relaxation by loosening up the muscles first in the face, and then in the eyes. Massaging your whole face influences the circulation around your eyes and teaches your brain not to tense up. Once you loosen this tension, it becomes much easier for the eyes to let go of tension, as well.

When you first begin your facial massage, spend at least a couple of minutes on each separate area, noticing how your touch feels and what effect it has. Breathe deeply, and try to connect with consciousness and care to this often-ignored part of your body. You may experience a deep tension or pain, a superficial tightness, a pleasant sense of release, or numbness (which is also a sensation).

Instructions

Rub your hands together until they are warm, and then massage your face with your fingertips—gently at first, and then more firmly as your muscles also begin to warm up. Initially, the pressure should be just firm enough to let you feel whether a spot is tense or painful, but not so hard that it makes the pain worse. Begin at the bridge of your nose, and move outward along the cheekbones, toward the temples. Stroke all the way along your cheekbones, from your nose to your ears. Feel the muscles in the area loosening under your fingers. Massage any sore spots, especially along the grooves of the muscles themselves, making circular movements with your fingertips and applying a little more pressure. Muscular tension will feel like hard, stringy, or fibrous spots under your fingers.

Now, from the bridge of the nose, work out along your eyebrows, massaging above, and directly on the brow. As you stroke, stretch the skin and underlying muscle very lightly. As you return to this stroking from time to time throughout your facial massage, gradually increase the amount of stretch to the skin and underlying muscles. Perform at least twenty strokes above the eyebrows and twenty on top of them as well. Avoid stroking below the eyebrow ridge.

Again, feel for grooves in your eyebrows while massaging. Massage these spots, making small circles with your fingertips. Sore spots are often found in the eyebrow area when there is eyestrain related to myopia, glaucoma, or retinal problems. They may occur above the bridge of the nose when one eye is dominant.

Spend a little extra time on the point between your eyebrows. This area gathers a lot of tension from the act of seeing. Then massage in long, firm strokes across your forehead and, very gently, with small circular motions, in the temple area (be careful not to press hard here). Stroke lightly from the temples up into your scalp, imagining that you are drawing tension away from your eyes.

Skin Rolling: The muscles on the forehead are more capable of tolerating a firmer massage than are other areas of the face, so we will begin here with a form of massage called *Skin Rolling.*

Begin by loosely pinching a fold of skin on the forehead with the thumb and fingers of both hands. Starting where it feels loosest, try rolling it along, up and down, and across your forehead. You can pinch the skin both vertically and horizontally as you move across your forehead. You can be vigorous with this massage. Try to feel that you are separating the skin and tense muscles from the skull.

Now, with a very soft touch, begin lightly stroking the eyelashes. The eyelashes are often neglected in self-massage, but softly stroking these tiny hairs can bring great relief to the eyelids. Breathe deeply, and imagine that these eyelashes do the work when you open and close your eyes. Allow your breath to deepen as you relax even further.

You can also expand the eye massage to the entire face and scalp. After skin rolling and massaging around the eye orbits, move into the jaw muscles, which habitually hold tension. Massage the whole area from the point of the chin outward along the jawbone, in front of and behind the ears. You can open and close your jaws while doing this, to help stretch and relax the strong jaw muscles. This may make you feel like yawning, so go ahead and yawn; it is very relaxing for your face. Massage your entire face, using one hand on either side and making large strokes from the midline outward.

Now move to your scalp. Grasp your hair and pull it gently, separating the skin and hair from your skull. Feel the circulation increasing, and breathe deeply to increase the circulation even more. Fan your hair out and let it fall from your hands.

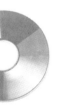

MORE INFORMATION ABOUT this exercise, and a guided version of this practice are included as tracks 5 and 6 of CD 1, Massaging and Moistening the Eyes, and Exercise Two: Facial Massage: A Preparation for Blinking

How often should I do this exercise?

Ideally, you should massage your face alone for at least 30 minutes in a given day. You can begin your day with a short massage before you go to work, with shorter massages throughout your day, and then end your day with a longer massage.

These massages are most beneficial when done in conjunction with all of the exercises.

Exercise Three: Blinking

Blinking is a natural massage for the eyes—it lubricates the eyes and also stops your vision for a short period of time, giving your eyes an immediate rest. When you blink, you momentarily stop light from coming into your pupils, and so dilate the pupils. When you give your pupils this rest, it increases their flexibility and makes it easier for them to respond to light.

When you use the computer, you may become so focused on what you see on the screen that you forget to blink. The average person blinks approximately twenty-two to twenty-three times per minute. When you use the computer, you only blink about six or seven times a minute. Therefore, it is a good practice to close your eyes from time to time throughout your day, and blink slowly and deliberately. The more you are aware of your blinking, the more you know when your eyes are tired, and that becomes a reminder for you to take a short break to blink, or to go outside and look far at a distance.

Eye tension, when it goes unchecked, can translate into other physical and mental tension, like stress about not meeting deadlines, tension with fellow workers, and a variety of other tensions. In addition, there is a cumulative effect of all of these tensions on our eyes and general stress level. However, if you take a few minutes out of your day to blink and soothe the eyes, it can reduce the amount of tension in your mind and body.

As you know by now, eye tension can lead to poor vision. Most people with bad eyesight have lost the ability to blink easily and often. When you see someone wearing thick glasses, you will notice that they tend to stare without blinking, and probably also frown and squint often. Dr. Bates once said that you can either squint or see well, but you cannot do both. The blinking exercises in this program will to help relax your squint and free your gaze to move fluidly from one object to another without freezing.

This is a simple but powerful exercise. Blinking:
- bathes and massages your eyes
- rests them from the work of focusing on near vision
- relieves tension around your eyes
- dismantles the harmful habit of staring

Instructions

Begin by slowly, gently opening and closing your eyes. Feel the lightness of your eyelids as you imagine that your eyelashes are doing the work of opening and closing the lids. Breathe deeply, and allow your breath to bring circulation into your eyelids, making them feel even lighter. Put your hand over your forehead as you blink, and make sure that it is not tense or frowning. If your forehead does not move, it means that your blinking is relaxed. If it does move, take some time to do some facial massage and skin rolling before resuming your blinking. Consult a mirror to make sure that you open and close your eyes fully with each blink—or check with a partner who is doing the eye exercises with you.

Now close your right eye and cover it with your right hand. Your fingers should be gently touching the closed eyelid. Begin slowly blinking your left eye. You can either imagine that the eyelashes are moving the eyelid up and down, with the eyelid merely an idle passenger; or you can picture someone gently raising the eyelid for you. Then release it so that gravity can pull it gradually down again. Brush the eyelashes of your left eye with the fingers of your left hand to reinforce the sense that they, and not your forehead, are doing the work. Try blinking so gently that the fingers of your right hand feel no movement in the right eyelid. This may take some time to accomplish; but the more you practice with this intention, the more both eyes will relax.

Now repeat the exercise, covering your left eye and blinking with your right eye.

A MORE IN-DEPTH guided version of this practice is included as track 7 of CD 1, Exercise Three: Blinking, and a track 5 of CD 2, Exercise Three Variation: Blinking

How Often Should I Do This Exercise?

As with all the other exercises in this program, blinking should be done with awareness and without strain. You should do this specific blinking exercise at least three times throughout your day. Try to let your blinking be effortless, frequent but not too rapid, complete but not forced. Try blinking instead of squinting when your eyes feel overwhelmed by bright light, since squinting not only tightens the muscles around the eyes, but also focuses light on the eyes in a painful and harmful way.

In addition to this specific exercise, you should also blink frequently throughout your waking hours. Blinking is a kind of a feedback mechanism to let you know that you may need to take a break and give your eyes a rest. You will be able to tell that it is time for a break when you begin to pay attention to how your eyes feel when you consciously decide to blink. If you begin to blink and notice that the eyes feel dry, that is the sign that your eyes need a break. Take a few moments throughout the day to check in with your eyes and blink them softly while you breathe deeply. Remember to blink frequently when you are doing a lot of near-field looking, as is the case when driving or working at a computer. In general, try to blink as often as you can throughout the day, and do the specific blinking exercises in the program at least three times a day. Doing so will increase your eye consciousness, and will be the quickest and most helpful tool in relieving your eye tension.

Exercise Four: Sunning

Sunning is a primary exercise for training your eyes to accept the light of day—a capacity many of us have lost after spending most of our lives indoors. Sunning helps us on many levels. First, Sunning helps to stimulate the *macula,* which is the central part of the retina, containing the specific cells which are sensitive to sunlight. Sunning also allows the pupils to become more flexible by contracting and expanding. When you Sun, you move your head from side to side and, even though your eyes are closed, your pupils respond to the change in light. When your eyes are closest to the strongest point of light, your pupils will contract, and when they are farthest away from the light source, they will expand. This contraction and expansion creates strength and flexibility in the pupils.

Finally, Sunning stimulates pigments in the *melanin layer* of the retina. These pigments darken the appearance of light to our eyes, which naturally protects them from sunlight. This process is similar to the effects of wearing sunglasses. Sunglasses, in fact, act as a kind of crutch for our eyes, and our pupils are prevented from adjusting to light naturally. When you put on sunglasses, the pupils become wide, and the pigments in the retina actually migrate away from the retina, because the light is not falling on the macula. This is why it is highly recommended not to wear sunglasses when you are out in the sun. While you never want to look directly into the sun, it actually strengthens your pupils when you allow your eyes to adjust to the varying levels of light naturally through the action of the pupil. This is also why it is important to learn the facial massage, so that you will not squint or tense up the muscles around the eye when you are out in bright sunlight.

Tips for Sunning

Always keep your eyes gently shut while practicing this exercise. Not even the healthiest eyes are equipped to tolerate intense light. The purpose of Sunning is to train your pupils to adapt readily to natural extremes of light and dark. Keep rotating your head or upper body continually through an entire 180-degree arc while Sunning to prevent retinal damage.

Never Sun through glass—either lenses or a window.
Any type of glass intensifies the sun's rays, which can damage your eyes.

Do this exercise at a time of day when the sunlight is coming into your eyes at a diagonal angle and is not too strong. Generally speaking, before 10:00 a.m. and after 4:00 p.m. are the ideal times to Sun; but this guideline can change in different regions and seasons. Use sunblock to protect your skin during the warmer seasons.

Do not sit still in the sun with your eyes closed. The side-to-side movement prescribed in Sunning is meant to create flexibility in the pupils. Sitting still under the sun allows too much light and radiation into the pupils.

If you began to feel headachy, nauseated, and/or dizzy, stop immediately and get out of the sun—it may be too bright for you, or you may be dehydrating.

If you find yourself having an uncomfortable sensitivity to light, do not Sun, and please see an ophthalmologist to ensure that you do not have an eye infection.

Instructions

Sit or stand outside or at an open window (remember: never Sun through glass). Close your eyes. Facing the sun, move your head from side to side, bringing your chin all the way to your shoulder before turning back to the other shoulder. Imagine that someone is holding your head between their hands and very gently turning it for you. Breathe deeply and slowly.

Your head should move:
• Constantly, without stopping
• As slowly as possible, as though it were rolling lazily from one shoulder to the other (chin to shoulder, not ear to shoulder)
• Effortlessly, a full 180 degrees (most people will need to move their whole upper body to complete the movement)

Turn from side to side in this way at least thirty times, relaxing your eyes as you do so. Imagine that the sun is bathing your eyes and head. Feel it penetrating all the way through your body. Sense the sun enveloping your head and brain; feel it penetrating to the back of your head, the back of your torso, the back of your legs.

Rub your hands together and, still rubbing, turn your back to the sun. Palm (*see Exercise Five*) for at least the duration of ten slow, deep breaths. Now turn back and sun again. Remember to keep breathing deeply and slowly. If you are comfortable with it, continue this alternation of approximately 2 minutes of Sunning with 1 or 2 minutes of Palming for up to 25 minutes.

You will probably notice a sense of relaxation in your eyes as they become accustomed to the bright light. You may also notice that the color you see while Sunning becomes brighter, while the color you see while Palming becomes progressively darker, until you are truly seeing perfect blackness. When this happens, you will know that the irises of your eyes have become more flexible, making the change from darkness to light with greater ease. Your optic nerve will be more relaxed, able to more comfortably receive stimuli, and more able to rest after receiving them.

When you have practiced Sunning for several weeks, you may gradually begin to Sun for longer periods—perhaps 5 or 6 minutes—between Palming interludes; but it is always a good idea to break up the Sunning with Palming. Not only does this give your eyes a rest, it also encourages flexibility in the irises.

Your eye muscles may resist the light at first, even with your eyes closed. Try to notice whether you sense tension in your eyes or around them, and allow the muscles to relax. Also notice the strength of the light coming though your closed lids, and the color of the light that penetrates your eyelids—this can range from dark red, through orange and yellow, to a brilliant white. If you see green, it means your eyes are straining. You should discontinue Sunning for a while, and try some Palming before returning to it.

MORE INFORMATION ABOUT this exercise, and a guided version of this practice are included as tracks 8 and 9 of CD 1, Creating Flexibility in the Pupils and Exercise Four: Sunning, and as tracks 6 and 7 of CD 2, Break Your Sunglasses Now! and Exercise Four Variation: Sunning

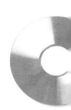

How often should I do this exercise?

Twenty minutes of Sunning per day is my average recommendation. You can break this down into sessions of 5 to 15 minutes, depending on how much your eyes have adapted to accept more light. Do not let your eyes become tired or strained; if they do, be sure to Palm until they feel good again. A cool cloth compress on your closed eyes is also very soothing and refreshing, especially on a hot day or in hot climates.

Note: After teaching and practicing Sunning with literally thousands of students, I have never known Sunning to damage anyone's eyes. Some doctors, however, believe that exposure to the sun can encourage the formation of cataracts. If this is of concern to you, please talk with your ophthalmologist about Sunning. If your doctor objects to the practice, inquire about studies proving the connection between eye damage and the sun. Take the time to read them yourself, and if you still feel uncomfortable about Sunning, please do not do it.

Sunning variation

After Sunning for about 10 minutes, try the following variation. Here, you will massage your eyebrows to increase the amount of light entering your eyes. Close your eyes, and place your right index and middle fingers on your right eyebrow, with your hand held high enough so that it does not block light from entering your right eye. Now turn your head slowly to the left, pressing gently but firmly upward with your fingertips as you do so. The motion of your head causes your fingers, which are stationary, to stroke your eyebrow. Your fingertips should exert a gentle pull on the eyebrow, stretching it. Your eye should remain closed.

Move your head all the way to the left, then to the right, and alternate several times. Then switch hands, placing the left index and middle fingers on your left eyebrow as your head turns to the right. This may take some practice to do smoothly. Remember to breathe deeply, move slowly, and relax. Repeat this motion several times, Palm (*see Exercise Five*), and return to the original Sunning.

Exercise Five: Palming

The purpose of Palming is to nurture your eyes in a deliberate and conscious way. Palming gives your eyes a rest in a way that even sleep does not. When you sleep, you are passive and are not in control of the visual images, mental activity, and rapid eye movement that occurs. When you Palm, you are focusing on relaxing your body, and resting your eyes as they experience a complete absence of light.

Palming is done with slow and deep breathing, relaxed shoulders, and—most importantly—completely relaxed hands. In fact, you should only do this exercise when your hands are relaxed, because you do not want to put tense or upset hands over your eyes. In some ways, palming is similar to energy massage or *Reiki* in that the heat and radiating energy of your hands can bring relief to tired and depleted eyes.

This supremely important exercise creates the relaxation that amplifies the effects of all the other exercises. It will:
- Rest the optic nerve
- Relax your nervous system
- Bring more circulation to your eyes

Tips for Palming
Never Palm with tense or upset hands. If your hands feel tense, take some time to breathe deeply, massage your hands, and relax before you Palm.

Never Palm with contacts in. Palming is meant to be a complete rest and relaxation for your eyes, and contacts do not allow the eyes to fully relax.

Instructions

Remove any jewelry from your fingers and wrists. Darken the room, and sit at a table with a cushion on it. Find a comfortable place to sit, and use pillows to prop up your elbows, since it allows your shoulders to relax more. Relaxing your shoulders will ensure that you do not put any pressure on your cheekbones or eye sockets. If you prefer, you can sit on the floor with your back against a wall and your elbows resting on your knees. It is also acceptable to lie down on your side, with your head and hand on a pillow. Support the other elbow with a second pillow. The proper posture allows you to hold your hands to your eyes without straining any part of your body, and without putting pressure on your eyes and face.

Warm your hands by rubbing them together, or by placing them on your chest, abdomen, or thighs. Drop your shoulders, and relax them by wiggling them for a moment. Close your eyes. Lightly rest the heels of your hands on your cheekbones, and cover your eyes with the palms of your hands. Your hands should not actually be touching your eyes.

Now start to imagine an ever-deepening blackness. As you progress with the Palming exercise, your optic nerve will relax, which will allow you to visualize an ever-increasing darkness. But to start, intend to see total blackness, and accept whatever you get. Do not try hard to eliminate all light, because this will put strain and effort on your Palming, which is ultimately counterproductive.

Visualize everything slowly turning black. If you wish, you can start with yourself. (If, for any reason, you are uncomfortable with the word "black," replace it in the following exercise with "dark," "darkness," or "midnight blue.") Imagine that your eyes themselves are black; or that your head is black. Continue until you can imagine your neck, chest, abdomen, thighs, knees, calves, and your feet are black themselves. Then imagine that all of the objects in the room are turning black, until the room is fully black. Imagine that the blackness is expanding beyond your room, into your building, and even beyond that, farther and farther outward, until the world itself is turning black. Feel free to create your own images of blackness. Relax into the meditation, enjoy giving free rein to your imagination, and notice how you feel.

At the same time, become aware of your breathing. Breathe deeply, slowly, and evenly through your nose. The more slowly you breathe, the better. Your exhalation should be slower than your inhalation.

While allowing everything to remain black, feel your abdomen and back expanding as you inhale, and shrinking as you exhale. Feel your chest, mid-back, and ribs expanding and shrinking as you breathe. Then feel your neck expanding and shrinking with each breath. (There is a gray area between sensation and visualization—just relax into it, and do not worry whether your neck is "really" expanding and shrinking.) Visualize or feel that your head is slowly expanding and shrinking with your breath, and that there is a slow, rhythmic movement of the bones of your skull as they move with your breathing.

Continue to breathe deeply, softly, pleasurably. Visualize that your pelvis is expanding and shrinking with your breathing, then your thighs, then your knees. Visualize that your fingers and toes are expanding and shrinking with your breathing. Notice how relaxed all these areas that you have breathed into are feeling now, including your eyes.

Now, while continuing to feel your body expanding and contracting with each breath, slowly begin to take away the blackness from the world outside, from your room, from your feet, on up through your body. When you feel ready, remove your hands from your eyes, and start to blink gently. If your eyes are watering, this is a good sign. Eyestrain tends to produce dryness, and watering is an indication that your eyes are genuinely relaxing.

While Palming, you may experience some of the painful, chronic eyestrain you have been shutting out. If you experience any discomfort in your eyes, continue to breathe and welcome the sensation until it passes.

The results of Palming differ widely from individual to individual. However much or little tension you have been able to release, continuing to practice Palming will lead to a lifetime of healthier eyesight.

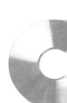

A GUIDED VERSION of this practice is included as track 10 of CD 1, Exercise Five: Palming, and as track 4 of CD 2, Exercise Five Variation: Palming

How often should I do this exercise?

It is impossible to Palm too many times or for too long—unless you have glaucoma or elevated pressure in the eyes. Otherwise, palm for at least 15 to 30 minutes, several times a day, for a minimum of 45 minutes in total.

Try to Palm at least twice a day, once before you begin your day, and once in the evening for a minimum of 20 minutes at a time, but preferably for 35 minutes in each sitting. It usually takes about 15 minutes to rest the eyes fully, and you should have at least a few minutes—more is better, naturally—to enjoy it. You should also try Palming in shorter segments, every 2 hours for 5 to 7 minutes per session, to help rest your eyes when taking a break from your work or reading. If you feel your vision problem is more serious, spend more time Palming.

If you suffer from glaucoma, restrict the Palming exercise to 4 or 5 minutes, or you may increase pressure in your eyes. You can, however, Palm briefly numerous times throughout the day.

Also, do not schedule a long Palming session just before you rush off on a million errands, because the chances are that you will not let yourself relax fully; nor is it wise to

Palm when you are extremely tired, unless your goal is to fall asleep immediately. Try to find a "between time," when you are neither exhausted nor anxious to get on to the next thing. Set aside a special time for Palming, and congratulate yourself if you go over the allotted time—it is a measure of how much you have been able to relax.

Emotional effects of Palming

You may experience a strong emotional resistance to palming, particularly if you palm and meditate at the same time. This is part of an overall resistance to relaxation that anxiety creates in many people. It is as though we believe that, if we let down our guard for a moment, disaster will strike from some unexpected quarter—and so we remain always slightly on edge: afraid of the dark, perhaps, or having difficulty relaxing with the natural sensations of being in your body.

If you find yourself overwhelmed by negative emotions, the best thing to do is try a meditative breathing exercise. This consists of ten deep breaths, drawn (as always) through your nose and deep into your abdomen. While you do this, give yourself permission to be exactly as you are. For these ten breaths, tell yourself that it is okay to be anxious, angry, or impatient; it is okay to have blurred vision. Tell yourself that whatever you think is wrong with you is not wrong; it just is. As you continue this meditative breathing, return to the Palming exercise.

Exercise Six: Stimulating Peripheral Vision

In primitive societies, people had a balanced use of their central and peripheral vision. They used both the *cone cells* of the eye—which are used for seeing fine detail and central vision—and the *rod cells,* which are used for seeing movement and peripheral vision. Today, the modern person mostly looks straight ahead, and does not look much with their periphery. When you read a book, work on the computer, or watch TV, you forget for hours at a time that you are surrounded by a world of other visual information.

Over time, you overuse the cone cells in the central vision, and the rod cells of the periphery start to become dormant. This leads to weakening of the macula—the area near the center of your retina—and can lead to poor vision and eyestrain. That is why it is very important to become more aware of your periphery by stimulating and strengthening it through eye exercises.

The exercises for peripheral vision will not only help stimulate the rod cells used for peripheral vision, but will also help create a more balanced use of the eyes by causing each eye to work independently, so neither eye can suppress what the other eye sees. When you learn to use your periphery more, you will also become much more relaxed and intuitive, because you will have more of an awareness of what is around you.

Instructions

The following exercise involves blocking your central field of vision and stimulating the periphery of each eye. To do this, you will need the three black pieces of paper (small, medium, and large) from the perforated strip included in your kit. These pieces of paper are used to block the central vision and to encourage your brain to pay attention to the visual information available within your periphery. If you should lose them, simply make your own by cutting out four pieces of black construction paper, all 2 inches in width. The first should be 1 ½ inches in length; the second 3 inches long; the third 6 inches long. Use a piece of double-backed adhesive tape—or regular masking tape doubled over—to stick the rectangle to the very top of the bridge of your nose. Keep these pieces of paper nearby for the following exercise.

Begin by sitting upright in a chair, covering your right eye with your right hand. Look straight ahead with your left eye while rotating your left arm, alternating in both directions all around your visual field. (The periphery of your left eye is not just to your left, but also above and below your face and to your right.). Remember to keep your gaze soft and focus straight ahead, not at the black paper itself.

As you look straight ahead, the movement in your arm stimulates the rod cells in your eye that pick up peripheral vision. Change sides, and cover your left eye with your left hand and move the right arm in a rotating motion as you look straight ahead.

Maintaining your gaze straight ahead, open both eyes and wave both arms to the side to stimulate your peripheral cells. Create a full circle by waving your arms in wide circles on both sides.

Now tape the smallest paper between your eyes. Look straight ahead at the paper while waving your hands and wiggling your fingers on both sides of your head, close to your ears. Vary the movement of your hands, moving them in circles, up and down, and out to the sides. Imagine that your peripheral field is expanding. To make sure you are using both eyes equally; always remember to pay conscious attention to what each eye is seeing.

To increase the stimulation to the periphery, begin to move your entire upper torso up and down, hinging at the hip while continuing to wave your hands and wiggle your fingers to the side. Imagine as you do so that the room, not your body, is moving opposite to your own movement. Thus, as your body moves downward, imagine that the room is moving upward; and as your body comes up again, imagine that the room is moving down. Breathe deeply and slowly as you do ten repititions of this movement.

Remove the small paper from between your eyes, and repeat this exercise with the mid-sized paper; then with the largest paper. After you have finished the up-and-down motion with the large paper, rub your hands together to warm them, and with the large paper still on the bridge of your nose, sit upright and palm for two full breaths.

Finally, repeat the exercise, using first the medium-size paper, and then the smallest paper. You will probably find, after this sequence, that your periphery has enlarged—and thus the smallest paper seems smaller than when you first used it.

MORE INFORMATION ABOUT this exercise, and a guided version of this practice are included as track 11 of CD 1, Exercise Six: Stimulating Peripheral Vision, and as tracks 8 and 9 of CD 2, Balancing the Eyes and Exercise Six Variation: Stimulating Peripheral Vision

How often should I do this exercise?

Repetition of this exercise at least once a day for 5 to 10 minutes is essential to improve your peripheral vision. If you are able, try to take a break from your day, and do the exercise three to four times a day for 2 to 3 minutes at a time, and it will make a huge difference in your vision.

Exercise Seven: Dominant Eye Test

The purpose of this exercise is to help you determine which eye is your dominant or strong eye. This is the eye that does the majority of the work when you look with both eyes. Ideally, you would not have a dominant eye, because both eyes would be working equally to see an object, but the majority of people have an eye that dominates. Unfortunately, once you develop a dominating eye, that eye will continue to dominate in all situations, and your other will become weaker over time.

Instructions

Fix your gaze on an object about one to three feet away from you, like a picture, a light switch, or a tree. Look straight ahead at that object with both eyes open, and put the thumb and fingers of both hands together creating a tunnel or hole through which you can see the object. Place your hands in the center of your face, between your eyes. Now, close one eye and see the object through your open eye. Notice how much of the object you can see with the open eye. Now close the other eye and look with that eye at the object. Notice how much of the object you can see with this eye. Continue to alternate between each open eye until you notice which eye allows you to see more of the object as a whole image.

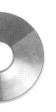

A GUIDED VERSION of this practice is included as track 12, Exercise Seven: Dominant Eye Test on CD 1

You may notice that the object simply shifts from right to left as you alternate between open eyes. If this occurs, make a smaller, rounder opening with your hands and fingers, so that the opening is about as large as a silver dollar. Look at the object again, first with both eyes, and then with each of your eyes individually. You should notice that you can see much more of the object with one of your eyes.

This eye is your dominant eye. Some of the exercises in this program require you to cover this eye in order to focus on strengthening the vision in your non-dominant eye, or weaker eye, creating a more balanced use of both eyes.

Shifting

The normal eye makes many tiny movements per second. These are known as *saccadic movements,* from *saccade,* the French for "jerk." You may have noticed that the eyes of people with exceptionally good vision often have a sparkling or piercing quality. This appearance is caused by these constant small movements of the eyes, which produce not only a special brightness, but also clarity and sharpness of vision. Whether the shifting is automatic or deliberate, the actual movement is invisible to the observer. Your eyes will simply look alert and lively.

The purpose of saccadic movements is to engage the macula, the part of the eye solely responsible for sharp, detailed vision. (The spot that sees with greatest clarity, the *fovea,* is in the center of the macula.) When we see with any part of the eye other than the macula, we lose most of our capacity for detailed vision. Because it is so small, the macula can see only small portions of the visual field at any one moment, although it sees them in very fine detail. For this reason, the normal eye makes constant, small, rapid movements as the macula moves from point to point, receiving a constant stream of visual information.

When vision begins to deteriorate, the saccadic movements become slower, larger, and less frequent. Vision blurs as details lose their definition or are lost altogether. This freezing of vision can arise from physical and/or emotional causes.

Shifting exercises are designed to restore the natural free movement of the macula. As the name implies, these exercises all involve shifting your point of focus from place to place, in imitation of normal saccadic movement. Though this movement must be consciously practiced at first, with time it becomes an automatic and effortless process, as it is for the healthy eye.

When you practice Shifting, the key to success is to maintain a soft focus. Allow yourself to see whatever you can see, without straining or forcing yourself to see anything in particular. Do not demand from yourself that you see any specific detail with clarity. Instead, allow your eyes and your mind to take in every detail available, without straining after those that are not yet available. If you do fixate on the point you are trying to see, your vision will freeze, and shifting will stop.

For anyone who wears glasses, no matter how strong or weak the prescription, a soft gaze is especially important. You have been accustomed to using your glasses to focus on whatever details you want to see. Now you must be willing to give this up—at least temporarily. Ironically, first you must give up your need to see clearly before you can improve your vision.

Your eyes may grow tired during Shifting—not because the Shifting itself is strenuous, but because you bring into it your old habits of straining to see. When this happens, take a break from Shifting for a moment or two. Palm, Sun, or close your eyes and visualize random and beautiful patterns of movement, such as waves rolling in, seagulls wheeling, or clouds blowing across the sky. Let your mind's eye move with these images for a minute or two, and then try to continue a graceful, easy flow of movement when you open your eyes and look again.

Exercise Eight: Shifting with Chart 1

Shifting with variously sized print teaches relaxed, strong focusing skills. Use Chart 1 for this exercise. Make sure you have removed your contact lenses or glasses. The key is to stay relaxed—your eyes work a lot better when you cut down on needless effort. Instead of straining to see, maintain a neutral state of mind, and allow what you are looking at to appear to you.

Instructions

Find a quiet spot, preferably a place where sunlight can fall on the page. Take Chart 1, with the differently sized print, and the small black piece of paper, and go outdoors into sunlight or a well-lit area. Face the sun, and do some sunning for about 2 minutes. Then take Chart 1 and hold it in your hand at a distance where you can read the largest row, but the letters are slightly fuzzy. If the largest row is very clear even when you hold the chart as far as you can away from your eyes, look at the next smallest row so that you can see the words, but the lines of the letters appear fuzzy.

Begin by looking at this row. Start to look at the print, one letter at a time. Let your gaze rest softly on the letters, and do not strain to see the detail. Let your eyes take a walk over each letter, feeling out its shape and the spaces around it. Your brain gets its focusing cues from edges, borders, and in-between spaces—you are giving it an extra nudge.

Now, look at the next smallest row. You will notice that it is harder to see the details, but do not strain to see the details; rather allow your gaze to rest softly on whatever you see. Do not try to read the letters, but accept the blurs, and let your eyes get curious and explore them—the blackness of the letters, the spaces between them. Work your way down the chart to the smallest row. At this point, stop the exercise and check whether your eyes feel tired. They often need a lot of relaxation when you are reprogramming visual habits. Take a few slow, deep breaths, relaxing into the out-breath.

Now close your eyes and breathe deeply as you visualize that the page is white and the letters are black. Breathe deeply as you visualize this. Now open your eyes and look at the smallest row of print. Consider the letters as if they were strange objects from outer space, investigating blackness, shapes, and the spaces between them. After looking at the smallest row, look back at the largest row and notice if you see the details of the letters any more clearly.

Now take the small piece of paper and tape it onto the bridge of your nose so that it covers your dominant eye, and wave your hand to the side of the covered (dominant) eye. While continuing to wave your hand to the side of the eye, look at the largest row. Then look at the next smallest row while continuing to wave your hand to the side. Continue this with the next smallest row and then the smallest row. Now, close your eyes and say in your mind, "The ink is black and the page is white," several times. Breathe deeply and slowly.

Now, look far at a distance with your non-dominant eye for several minutes, and allow your eye to rest as you do this. Now look at the largest row of print. You will most likely notice that the print is much clearer. Take off the piece of paper, and look at the largest row with both eyes—the row should be clearer.

A GUIDED VERSION of this practice is included as track 13 of CD 1, Exercise Eight: Shifting with Chart 1

How often should I do this exercise?
When you are using your computer, you can look at this chart from time to time to measure the condition of your

eyes. When you notice that the page is becoming blurry, take 20 minutes out of your day to do this exercise.

Exercise Thirteen: Shifting with Chart 1 and Chart 2

Instructions

Take Chart 1, Chart 2, the small, medium, and large pieces of paper, and a brightly colored ball or a tennis ball outside in the bright sun or into a well-lit area outdoors. Attach Chart 2 to a tree, fence, or post, and stand at a distance where you can read at least the top three lines, but you cannot read the bottom three lines.

Now, take Chart 1 and hold it in your hand at a distance where you can read the largest or next largest row, but the letters are slightly fuzzy.

Now that you have established the proper distances, make a mental note of how far away you are holding Chart 1, and then turn away from the sun and do some Sunning for about 3 minutes. Relax and breathe deeply. After 3 minutes of Sunning, turn away from the sun and do one minute of Palming.

Now turn to the sun and do 3 more minutes of Sunning. Slowly open your eyes and look at Chart 2, the standard eye chart, and see how the letters appear to you. You may notice that you can read an additional line. Look at Chart 1. You may see that the lines are less fuzzy.

Turn around, away from the sun, and look far at a distance for 1 minute, waving your hands to the side to relax your eyes and stimulate your peripheral vision.

Now turn back toward Chart 2 and tape the small piece of paper so that it completely obstructs your dominant eye. Wave your hand to the side of the strong eye as you look at Chart 2, and see which row looks most clear to you before it becomes fuzzy. Do not try to read the letters. Let your eyes get curious and explore them—the blackness of the letters and the spaces between them.

Continue with this until you have done this for all of the rows, down to the smallest row. Once you have finished looking at the smallest row, close your eyes and say to yourself, "The ink is black, the page is white." Open your eyes and look at the largest row that you began with. Does it look any more clear? The more time you spend doing this exercise, the more your eyes will feel relaxed and alive. In bad weather, do this exercise indoors. You can substitute Palming for Sunning to reduce your eyestrain.

A GUIDED VERSION of this practice is included as track 14 of CD 2, Exercise Thirteen: Shifting with Chart 1 and Chart 2

How often should I do this exercise?
When you begin to work on your eyes, you should do this exercise once a day for at least 20 minutes at a time. Your aim is ultimately to make Shifting an automatic function.

Exercise Nine: Long Swing
The purpose of this exercise is to increase the sense of movement while you are engaged in the act of seeing. Practiced regularly, the long swing will:
- break up the habit of straining to see
- stimulate your peripheral vision
- integrate the field of vision (especially helpful for people with low visual capability)

Instructions
Stand with your legs wider than hip width, about 2 feet, apart. Hold up a finger about 10 inches in front of your nose, and look at it. Keep looking at your finger while you move your torso from side to side, turning so that your finger is always in front of your nose. As you look at your finger, notice that everything seems to move in the opposite direction, as if you were looking out of a moving train. From time to time, stop the active exercise, close your eyes,

and visualize what you just saw: your finger moving in one direction and everything else moving in the opposite direction. Then resume the active exercise.

Now, hold your finger horizontally rather than vertically, and move up and down, hinging at your hips and following the movement of your finger with your eyes and head, just as you did in the vertical direction. As you move your face up, everything will seem to move downward, an so on. Keep moving up and down, breathing deeply and slowly, and blinking. You may find it easier to see things moving in the opposite direction to your own motion. End by Palming for a moment.

Variation: You can do a variation of this by combining the horizontal and vertical long swings into a U-shaped long swing (it is also a nice workout!). Hold your finger vertically again. Always looking at the finger and keeping it in front of your nose, stretch tall as you pivot to the left, swoop down into a forward bend in the middle of your arc, and then stretch tall again as you pivot to the right. (Note: Some people like to change the fingers at the midpoint. Try both ways, and use whatever method works best for you.) You may even want to throw your head back and arch your back a little at the left and right ends of the arc.

A GUIDED VERSION of this practice is included as track 14 of CD 1, Exercise Nine: Long Swing

How often should I do this exercise?
Do this exercise two to three times a day throughout your day for 3 to 5 minutes at a time. You can do it before you begin work, again during lunch, and before you go home. It is a wonderful way to demonstrate to the brain and body that your eyes can see in a balanced way without straining.

Relaxing Your Body

Circulation is a very important aspect of eye health. Many of the eye and body problems today are a result of poor circulation, which can also cause serious pathologies, such as glaucoma. Studies have shown that men who wear neckties have more tension and more incidents of glaucoma related to restricted circulation to the head. A group of optometrists who did an experiment with thirty-one people showed that light exercise brings more circulation to the eye and measurably lessens pressure in the eyes. There are also studies that show that increased blood circulation to the head can help prevent stress and slow the aging process.

It is impossible to relax one part of your body—your eyes, for example—if other parts of your body are tense. Therefore, it is helpful to begin each exercise with some elementary body relaxation exercises. To get the best results, it is preferable if you can find a place on the floor where you can sit and lie down comfortably. Feel free to use a blanket or a mat if it helps you.

Exercise Ten: Shoulder and Back Release

Instructions

As with all of the exercises described in this program, you should breathe slowly and deeply, through your nose. This action helps you to relax both physically and mentally, while it also enriches your blood with the oxygen your eyes need to function at their best.

First, find a comfortable sitting position. Sit upright with your spine erect, and breathe deeply into your belly. Now interlace your fingers above your head, with your palms pointed toward you. Rotate your arms in a large circle, reaching as far as you can without straining. Do a few circles clockwise and another few counterclockwise. This exercise is wonderful for releasing shoulder and upper-back tension, since they work directly on the shoulder muscles. If you have ever had these muscles massaged, you know how tight they can get. Allow all of the tension in your shoulders to relax and melt away.

Now begin to tap lightly on the tip of the left shoulder with your right hand. Continue to tap as you rotate the left arm in a clockwise circle. Then change directions and rotate your left arm in the opposite direction. Next, tap lightly on the tip of the right shoulder with your left hand. As you tap, rotate your right arm, first clockwise, and then counterclockwise.

Next, find a comfortable position lying on your right side with your knees bent. Use a pillow to support your head and keep your spine in proper alignment. Use your left arm to stabilize yourself if necessary, and move the tip of your shoulder in a rotating motion as if you were shrugging. Imagine that the tip of the shoulder is doing the work as you move the shoulder clockwise and then counterclockwise. Now, move your entire left arm in a rotating motion, first clockwise and then counterclockwise.

Switch sides. Lie on your left side and begin to rotate the tip of your right shoulder in a shrugging motion. Rotate in one direction and then move it in the opposite direction. Then move your entire right arm in a rotating circular motion, as widely as your shoulder will allow. Do not force this motion, but rather let gravity do the work as you gently stretch your shoulder, abdomen, and back. Now rotate your arm in the opposite direction.

More information about this exercise, and a guided version of this practice are included as tracks 2 and 3 of CD 2, Activating Relaxation, and Exercise Ten: Shoulder and Back Release

Exercise Twelve: Back and Neck Release

Instructions
Sit cross-legged on the floor, with your right calf in front of your left calf. Sit upright with your spine erect, and breathe

slowly and deeply. Hold your knees with your hands, and move your entire upper body in a rotating motion. Move evenly to the side, back, side, and front. Make sure your neck and chin are relaxed, but comfortably stretched. Now move in the opposition direction with a slow and smooth movement to the side, back, side, and front.

Change the position of your legs so that your left calf is in front of the right calf. Hold your knees with your hands, and move in a rotating motion, first in one direction for a few rotations, and then in the opposite direction. Breathe slowly and deeply, and allow your body to relax.

The next exercise is designed to help loosen any tension that may be built up in your neck and back. Move onto your knees and hands, and lean forward so that your forehead is touching the floor. Use your forehead as a pivoting point, and rotate your head from side to side, allowing your neck to remain long and relaxed. Imagine that your chin or forehead is directing the movement. Use your hands to modify the pressure so that you are not bearing too much weight on your forehead.

Once you are comfortable with this movement, you can move farther forward onto the crown of your head, and move your head in a rotating motion to allow for a deeper neck and back release. Breathe deeply and slowly.

Move into a cross-legged position again, hold your left knee with both hands, and stretch your entire torso toward your knee. If you want to increase your stretch, first stretch backwards, away from the knee, and then move the entire torso forward, toward your knee. Move your head slightly toward the knee, but be careful not to create too much of an arch in your back as you do this. This exercise is meant to help release tension in your back and neck.

Now hold your right knee with both hands, and first stretch away from the knee in the opposite direction, then bend the entire torso toward the knee. Breathe deeply and slowly. Finally, stretch your hands down the center of your crossed legs, and allow your neck and back to release into this stretch as you bend forward with your entire torso.

Now sit upright with your legs still crossed, and move your upper body in a rotating motion, first in one direction and then in the opposite direction.

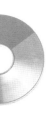

MORE INFORMATION ABOUT this exercise, and a guided version of this practice are included as tracks 12 and 13 of CD 2, Increasing Circulation to the Eyes, and Exercise Twelve: Back and Neck Release

How often should I do this exercise?

These exercises are best done before you do any of the longer eye exercises, like Palming or Sunning. These exercises help you to create the relaxation in the neck, middle back, and shoulders that is necessary to do the other exercises. Take as much time as you need to do these exercises in order to fully alleviate your tension.

Exercise Eleven: The Melissa Exercise

The Melissa exercise entails separating the two eyes with a strip of paper and throwing a ball from one hand to another. Sounds easy enough, right? Not always so. As you know from the Dominant Eye Test (*see Exercise Seven*), you probably have one eye that works a little bit harder than the other—an imbalance in your vision that can lead to eyestrain and poor vision.

This exercise specifically works on creating a more balanced use of both eyes. To create this balance, you will learn to use your eyes independently of each other. This exercise also helps teach the body and the brain that, even when your eyes must work independently of each other, you can still see and function. When you take the ball and throw it from hand to hand, you physically respond to a new concept. In the thalamus, there is connection between the sense of touch and the sense of sight, connecting to

66

receptors in the brain. When you do this exercise, you strengthen that connection.

Teaching the brain and body this simple exercise will improve your vision. When you separate the eyes from each other and integrate exercises that require hand/eye coordination for both the right and left eyes independently, you will strengthen each eye independently. Later, when your eyes work together, they will be more balanced.

Do not be discouraged if you keep dropping the ball. The reason you will drop the ball is that you are accustomed to having more control with your dominant eye. Most people's sense of control is visual, so as soon as you put the paper between your eyes, you will lose that sense of control to some degree. Momentarily feeling out of control is actually good for you, because your usual sense of being in control involves maintaining your ingrained habits through a considerable amount of tension.

It may take several weeks—or even several months—until this exercise seems easy to you. However, the real point of this exercise is to get your two eyes to work together, and to build new patterns and habits of seeing that will eventually lead to a new, balanced way of seeing.

Instructions

Take the longest (non-perforated) piece of paper and use the masking tape to tape it down the center of your face, from your forehead to your chin. Stand up, take a brightly colored ball or a tennis ball, and throw it from one hand to the other. The ball should be thrown in such a way that it goes a few inches above your head when thrown from one hand to the other. Keep your head fixed and facing straight ahead, and follow the ball with your eyes as you throw the ball from one hand to the other. There should be a brief moment when the sight of the ball will disappear from your visual field as it rises above the height of your head.

Take your time as you do this exercise, and remember to breathe deeply. Make sure your neck is loose.

When you can perform this part of the exercise comfortably, continue to throw the ball from one hand to the other as you begin to walk very slowly forward. If you are doing this indoors, take small steps, or find a hallway or large room where you will not run into anything. As you walk, you may find that it is actually easier to throw and catch the ball, as you are integrating more of your body movement into the exercise.

If you want to add an additional element to this exercise, close alternating eyes. For example, as you throw the ball to your right hand, close your left eye. Then, when you throw the ball to your left, close the right eye. In this way the side that is receiving the ball has the open eye and the side that is throwing the ball has the closed eye. When you get better at this exercise, you can even begin to walk slowly forward as you do this.

Remember, the goal of this exercise is to create a balanced use of your eyes; it is not to be successful at throwing and catching the ball. If you are attempting to throw the ball from one hand to the other while following it with your eyes, you are already successful!

A GUIDED VERSION of this practice is included as track 11 of CD 2, Exercise Eleven: Melissa Exercise

How often should I do this exercise?

Do this exercise 10 minutes a day, every day, starting with the basic exercise of throwing the ball from one hand to the other while walking. Then, as you get better, you can close alternating eyes, and eventually again add in walking as you do this. If you are diligent and patient with yourself, you will create a more balanced use of your eyes, and notice a significant decrease in the dominance of your strong eye.

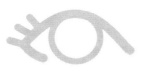

Chapter Eight

Other Exercises You Can Do

Neck and Shoulder Relaxation

Close your eyes and let your face go slack, especially around the jaw, which tends to tense automatically with deep concentration. Turn your head to the side and gently feel with your fingertips along the side of your neck. The *sternocleidomastoid muscle* runs from underneath your ear, down along the side of your neck, and into the breastbone and collarbone. This muscle bears much of the burden for supporting the head, and so relaxing its tension is vital to the health of your eyes. The sternocleidomastoid can become tighter than just about any other muscle in your body (some people have mistaken it for a bone when touching it), so give it a lot of special attention.

Massage all along the length of this muscle, trying to follow the path of tension. Palpate, tap, and stroke it—gently at first, and then more firmly as it begins to soften. You will probably find several very sore or tight spots. Do not dig at them, because they are probably so sore that they will only resist deep massage. Instead, work gently on them and more firmly around them. Now turn your head from side to side, and see whether you notice a difference between the two sides. Notice any difference in muscle tension, and then massage the other side.

Next, imagine that someone is holding your head and moving it for you, so that it rolls very slowly and gently from side to side. Let it roll far enough to each side that you feel the stretch in the side neck muscles, jaw, and shoulders.

After practicing this movement until your neck begins to relax, slowly begin to open your mouth. Let it stretch as far as it can without strain, and then let it fall closed as you continue to roll your head from side to side. Pay attention to which muscles are moved by this exercise: where, besides the jaw, can you feel the stretch?

As you continue to roll your head and open and close your mouth, add a steady, rhythmic blinking. This is also a great coordination exercise, because you will have your head, jaw, and eyelids all moving at the same time, but at slightly different speeds. If you find this difficult, concentrate not on the difficulty, but on the different sensations that each part is experiencing as it moves. Do this for several minutes, and see whether you experience a sense of relief from facial and eye tension. If not, see whether you at least experience the tension itself. Many people carry this tension with them all the time, but never actually feel it. Nonetheless, it may eventually result in deteriorated eyesight.

When you have released some of the tension in your neck muscles, you are ready to do some head rotations. It is important to relax the neck first, as moving your head in this way with a tight neck can make you dizzy or nauseated. Rotate your head slowly, making relatively small circles. If you are doing this movement lying down, you do not have to lift your head to make a full rotation. Imagine that you are drawing a circle with your chin or nose; this will produce the correct motion.

You may be tempted to begin with huge, sweeping circles, trying to shake out the tension you feel in your neck and shoulders. The problem with this is that your body, when it feels that tension, interprets the movement as stress and resists it; so begin with small circles.

Touch the highest vertebra you can reach, where your skull and neck are joined, and imagine this as the center of the circle your head is making. This gentle motion not only relaxes your neck muscles, but also releases tension in your spinal joints, making movement of your neck more easy and fluid. Make at least one hundred of these slow, small rotations, and do not forget to change direction from clockwise to counterclockwise after every ten or fifteen circles.

Palming Sequence for Work

Before you start your day, stretch and do a good 15 minutes of Palming at home. When you get to work, go outside and look at clouds or something far in the horizon for about 7 minutes as you wave your hands to the side. Then massage around your eyes to relax them.

As you work at the computer during the day, pause every 10 minutes to Look Far at a Distance for 30 seconds at a time. This is the amount of time it will take your lens to flatten and relax. If possible, find a window at midmorning and Look Far at a Distance for about 2 minutes, and then sit down at your desk and Palm for another 4 minutes. Then put the piece of paper between your eyes and wave both hands to the side to stimulate your periphery. Do this with each size paper included in this set. Begin with the smallest size, and then continue with the medium and then the large sheet for about 1 minute each, palming between each size. When you have finished with the large piece, move back to the medium, then finally the small piece of paper, again for 1 minute each. If the small paper looks smaller, you will know that you have improved your peripheral vision.

Before lunch, stand up and do the Long Swing exercise for about 2 to 3 minutes, then go outside and look far at a distance for 7 to 10 minutes, adding in some Palming every 2 to 3 minutes.

When you are finished with your day, give yourself 5 to 7 minutes of continuous palming, making sure to breathe deeply as you relax your neck, shoulders, and hands. Finish the day by going outside and Looking Far at a Distance for about 5 to 7 minutes before you get into your car and drive home.

Using Broken Sunglasses or Glasses

Many of the exercises can be done while wearing frames from sunglasses or eyeglasses that have had the lenses removed and the side of the dominant eye taped over. For example, while wearing the glasses, take a brightly colored ball or a tennis ball, and either throw and catch it by yourself, or throw and catch with a partner. The obstruction over the dominant eye will help you see better with your non-dominant eye. You can do this exercise 15 minutes per day.

You can also do a combination of The Long Swing and Looking Far at a Distance using the glasses. Begin by Looking Far at a Distance for 3 minutes, then take the glasses off and Look Far at a Distance with both eyes for 3 minutes. Repeat the exercise with the glasses on, obstructing your dominant eye for 3 more minutes. Once again, take the glasses off and follow with 3 minutes of The Long Swing. You will notice your vision improving after doing this sequence.

Periphery Exercises

As long as you are not the driver, you can turn a car ride into a vision exercise by taping a rectangle of black paper onto the bridge of your nose. Look straight ahead at it; your brain will quickly tire of the black paper, and will begin paying more attention to the moving scenery on both sides. If you are on a train, try sitting so that you are facing the opposite direction to the one in which the train is moving. This will make you even more aware of the movement.

You can also do your computer work with the small piece of paper taped to the bridge of your nose to separate your eyes and cause them to work independently. If you do this, you will stretch your external eye muscles and give your dominant eye a rest, because it will not have to work as hard. When you have the paper between your eyes, throughout your workday, periodically look up with your eyes, then look down. You will use different eye muscles when you do this, and it will strengthen your overall vision.

Balancing the Muscles Around Your Eyes

The first technique is designed to increase the flexibility and strength of the muscles around your eyes, and teach them to move with equal ease in all directions.

Begin by moving both eyes simultaneously in small circles. If you find this difficult to do, you can hold up a finger in front of your eyes and move it in a circle, allowing the eyes to follow it; it is preferable, however, to rotate your eyes without this aid. Also move your eyes from side to side and up and down. If you find any position especially difficult, work gently with it by moving your eyes from side to side (or up and down) from that position.

As you do this exercise, touch your forehead above the eyes with your fingertips. Can you feel the muscles moving? They do not need to. Try to relax them, and practice this exercise until you can do it without working your forehead muscles. You may simply need to make your circles smaller; in fact, see how small you can make them. Now close your eyes, and visualize them moving in circles, freely, with no effort. It may help to picture a wheel rolling, or a record on a turntable. Open your eyes and rotate them again, this time imagining that only the pupils are rotating. Next, close your eyes and move them in a circle under the closed lids. This may be more difficult, since the movement is so much more limited. Touch your eyelids lightly as you do this, feeling the movement beneath them. Notice whether you tense the rest of your face during this motion; if so, try not to. You will find it much easier to do this exercise with your eyes open after this.

Shifting Exercises

Whenever you remember to, move your eyes from point to point on whatever it is you are looking at. Instead of looking at a tree, look at the individual parts that make up the tree, and then move from larger to smaller details of those parts. Remember to blink and breathe as often as possible; both of these actions will help your eyes to move more freely and easily. You may be surprised at the amount of detail you can see. Without necessarily gaining any measurable change in your vision, you will see better simply because you are seeing consciously.

Refine this process by taking note of those details you cannot see clearly. For example, you may be able to clearly distinguish a tree, a branch on the tree, and an individual leaf on the branch; but you may not be able to see the veins and markings on the leaf. Let your eyes roam freely over the leaf, noting whatever you can of its shape, color, and so on—anything that is available to your vision. Do not worry about forming an exact picture of the leaf. Just look at it, like a visitor from outer space who is seeing a leaf for the first time. Do not force yourself to see; just allow yourself to look. Then close your eyes, recall whatever details you can, and picture them in sharp contrast to their background. See the leaf as bright where the background is dark; in color where the background is white; coming toward you as the background recedes; or whatever will most sharply distinguish the object from its surroundings.

Bring fine details closer to you, making them more accessible. Take a picture that you like, and hold it close enough to see every detail clearly without straining; then shift from point to point. If you are looking at a face, hone in on one eye, and look at every separate eyelash, every separate spot of color in the iris. Divide the forehead into quarters, then into eighths, and so on, until you are looking at the smallest possible unit of detail. Close your eyes and recall those details you have seen, then open them again and look for new details.

After a while, you may notice the distinctions between separate details growing sharper. For some people, this change can happen almost instantaneously, while for others it takes months. The time factor is not important. Learning to see details is.

Reading

Typically, the first indication of some eye problems will occur when you notice that you have to alter the distance at which you need to hold a book in order to read comfortably. To determine your visual acuity, the eye doctor will ask you to read rows of printed letters on eye charts.

Reading is one of the most sensitive issues for a nearsighted person. The typical nearsighted person (and there is such a thing) loves to read, and would do it until their eyes gave out completely if time and life allowed. What few of us book-lovers remember is that reading is a strenuous physical activity involving a delicately balanced pair of organs. We become absorbed by the flow of information from the page to our minds, and forget how hard our eyes are working to create that flow.

Reading can potentially be very harmful for the eyes, which are biologically designed to adjust from close to distant focus continually. Reading does not have to be damaging, however; in fact, you can actually use reading to improve your overall vision. Reading exercises stimulate the habit of shifting, making them especially helpful for myopia, astigmatism, and hyperopia and presbiopia.

Protecting your eyes when you read
Most often, it is not the act of reading itself, but our poor reading habits that are responsible for the damage reading can do. Here are some general rules that will help make even prolonged reading easier for your eyes:

Look Far at a Distance for 7 minutes at a time before reading. Then, before you sit down to read, massage your eyes and wave your hands to the side.

Never read in uncomfortable light, whether too bright or too dim. The wrong light will tire your eyes faster than anything else. Your eyes will tell you if the light is wrong; all you need to do is pay attention to them. If reading feels difficult, the light is the first thing to check.

Just as you would naturally take breaks from hard physical labor, you need to give your eyes breaks from the hard labor of reading. At least every 20 minutes or so, stop and palm for about 5 minutes.

Blink constantly to keep your eyes from staring or drying out. If your eyes burn during or after reading, it may be because you become so involved with what you are reading that you forget to blink. Remind yourself to blink as often as you can.

As much as possible, avoid anything that is printed in a hard-to-read typeface. Many publications are printed in type so faint, so small, so unclear, so dense, or so elaborate that it would give anyone eyestrain. Stay away from such print. If you have difficulty with necessary reading tasks, such as legal documents or phone books, do not strain your eyes; read them when your eyes are rested, and in a comfortable light.

Breathe. Even though your mind may be in another world, your body is still in this one, and your eyes need oxygen more than ever. There is a tendency to hold one's breath while reading—as in many concentrated activities—so remind yourself to breathe as often as you remind yourself to blink.

Reading and Shifting

Speed reading, if you do it frequently, may eventually cause vision loss. In speed reading, you try to take in whole sentences—or even whole paragraphs—simultaneously. This behavior unconsciously imitates the pattern of myopic sight: making large, infrequent jumps and trying to take in a large visual field. Remember that the macula can see only small areas at a time, and that it sees by moving from point to point. Forcing your eyes to swallow an entire sentence at one gulp makes it impossible for the macula to participate fully—and, of course, the less your macula works, the more blurred your sight will be. (Shifting with Chart 1 may help you see details better and sharpen your eyesight.)

Reading upside down

Take this page, turn it upside down, and read one letter at a time, letting your eyes move from point to point as they slowly and carefully trace the shape of each letter. Blink constantly as you do so. This practice will train you to be more aware of the letters, focusing on the physical act of seeing rather than on the meaning of the words. It will also make you more aware of what your eyes are doing when you read—an awareness we usually lose in our absorption with the contents of a book. If you find this difficult, it is a clue that this is an especially effective exercise for you.

Reading and peripheral vision

When you read, write, or do any kind of work that could tax your central vision, it is very helpful to stimulate your peripheral vision by waving or wiggling your hands to the sides of your eyes. This motion genuinely takes the strain out of reading.

We have many opportunities to overwork our central vision and neglect the periphery: crowded city streets, narrow freeway lanes, computers, documents covered with tiny print and incomprehensible data—all these seem designed to promote tunnel vision and to narrow our horizons. Peripheral exercises are one way to counteract this problem.

Creating Flexibility Between Near and Distant Vision

Find yourself a pleasant place from which you can see well into the distance. The top of a hill or any other high place is especially useful. Look all the way to the farthest horizon, and let your eyes move from point to point, as though you are sketching the outlines of what you see. You may be able to distinguish only general shapes, colors, and degrees of brightness at this distance. Let your eyes enjoy playing with these, as they might enjoy looking at an abstract painting. Then focus your attention slightly closer, and keep your eyes shifting from point to point. Perhaps the details you see may be a bit more distinct, but remember not to become fixed on them or try too hard to see them. Just enjoy them, keeping your eyes soft and receptive. Repeat this process, bringing your plane of focus a little closer to you each time, until your eyes are shifting on the area immediately in front of you: on the windowsill, a heap of leaves on the ground, or your feet. At this point, look for the tiniest details you can possibly distinguish. Always remember to blink, breathe, and keep your focus soft as you do this and all eye exercises. Now repeat the exercise in reverse, choosing gradually more distant visual targets. Repeat the entire exercise several times.

Skying

The purpose of Skying is similar to that of Sunning: to teach your eyes and brain to accept light comfortably, without a sense of strain. It is a good alternative to Sunning on cloudy days.

Turn away from where the sun should be, in case it comes out again, and face the sky with eyes open. Blink continuously. Place one hand on the back of your head and the other on your forehead, making sure that the hand on your forehead does not block the light coming into your eyes. The hand on the back of your head should be curved into the shape of a claw, and the other stretched, with the bony prominences at the base of your fingers pressing hard on your forehead. Now move your head from side to side while keeping your hands in their original position. Only your head is moving; not your hands. As you turn your head, it should move against your hands, creating the effect of a firm massage to the back of your head and forehead. Doing this for several minutes will increase circulation and relaxation in your face, neck, and eyes. Palm for a minute, then return to the basic sunning exercise.

Night Walks

This exercise is similar to Sunning in that it helps create more flexibility in the pupils by allowing them to expand and contract with different light stimuli. Set aside time when you can walk for about 40 minutes outside at night. Bring along a stopwatch or watch that has a lighted screen, so you can see the time.

You can begin by dimming or completely turning off the lights where you are, and Palming for about 10 minutes. Then go outside in a neighborhood or park where you feel safe at night, and begin walking. After about 5 minutes of walking, put the small piece of paper on the bridge of your nose and walk for about one minute. Take the paper off and walk for another 10 minutes. Then repeat this practice, but before you put on the paper, stop walking and do the Long Swing exercise to create a sense of more light. You may begin to notice more detail in the stars and moonlight. Repeat this sequence every 10 minutes—Long Swing, walking for 1 minute with the small piece of paper on the bridge of your nose, then walking for 10 minutes, until about 40 minutes has passed. You will notice that it will appear much lighter outside, you will see greater contrast between light and dark, and the details of what you see will become more clear.

Testing Your Vision

Your progress with Natural Vision Improvement depends entirely on your own efforts and observations. There is no outside "expert" empowered to measure your progress and pronounce whether your condition is improving, and by how much. It is up to you to mark your starting point—much as a parent might mark a child's height on a doorjamb—and then to return from time to time to measure your improvement against that first mark.

The traditional way to test vision is with an eye chart, such as Chart 2, which is included with *The Natural Vision Improvement Kit.* For those of us who have spent more than our fair share of time in ophthalmologists' offices, however, the very sight of a regular eye chart can be stressful enough to freeze our eyes in panic. If this sounds familiar, create your own chart. Use drawings, pictures cut out of magazines, dried flowers, or symbols that have special meaning for you.

The only requirement is that, as in a traditional eye chart, you make all the items in the top row the same size; then create a second row of smaller items—again, all of the same size; and so on, with each row getting progressively smaller until you have six lines.

Hang your chart several feet away from you, at a distance where you can read one to three lines easily, but you have difficulty with the rest. The chart should be vertical (e.g., on a wall, rather than angled on a chair or easel), at a comfortable eye level for you, either when standing or sitting. Begin "reading" your chart at the top line. Make a note of the last line you can see clearly.

This is the yardstick against which you will measure your progress as you continue to practice Natural Vision Improvement. After each exercise—or at least after each session—return to your chart, standing the same distance away from it, and check for changes.

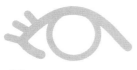

Chapter Nine

Optimizing Your Work Environment

If you are like most people, you will undoubtedly spend many hours a day in a work environment that causes you to look near at a computer, at text, or some other form of near-field vision. Here are some helpful tips for optimizing your work environment:

If you use a computer, use a glare screen to help minimize the glare and radiation effects on the eye.

If you focus on text, a computer, or anything else in the near field, adjust the lighting to create more contrast and illuminate what you are focusing on, but try to avoid overlighting your entire work space. You do not want to go to extremes here, as you still want to pick up movement that occurs in the periphery so you can continually be aware of it, but you want to create a contrast for the near-field vision so you do not strain to see the details. The proper level of lighting depends on how detailed your vision is. If you have excellent vision, a well-lit room is appropriate, but if you have poor vision, a semi-dark room will create the contrast to see details better.

If you wear contacts, keep your contact solution and case nearby so you can easily take your contacts out to do the exercises.

Keep a pillow nearby so you can easily use it to do the Palming exercises.

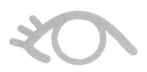

Conclusion
Making Time for Your Eyes

Dr. Bates was often asked, "Why do eye exercises take so long to do?" His answer was that we work on our eyes, one way or another, all the time. We either work on them in a way that freezes them, or we work on them in a way that makes them more alive. His suggestion was to take the opportunity to make our eyes more alive.

The most important step you can take, psychologically, is to decide that working on yourself and your eyesight is important. Modern life continuously assaults our eyes; thus the sign of a healthy psyche is that you are naturally moved to take care of them. The more common approach of simply doing whatever is expedient to make your eyes function points to a deeper problem: a commitment to achievement at all costs.

The happiness you seek through accomplishments is more readily available to you when you let go of meeting outside expectations, and begin to pay attention to what your mind, body, and spirit actually need. Paradoxically, you are likely to discover that the most important achievements of your life come relatively easily when you are truly taking care of yourself.

Because they are among the hardest-worked and least-nurtured organs in your body, your eyes are an excellent place to begin a program of self-care. Declare your intention to take care of your eyes all day long, and learn how much better you can feel—not only physically, but in every other way as well. Let your eyes teach you how to gradually change the way you look at the world—literally—so that well-being becomes more important to you than all the trophies this world can give you.

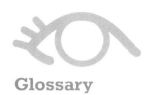

Glossary

Accommodation: Unconscious process by which the eye adjusts itself to focus on near objects. Accommodation is the work of autonomic muscles within the eye called the *ciliary muscles,* which contract, allowing the lens to become rounder. At rest, the eye is focused for distant vision, and the lens is relatively flat.

Astigmatism: Irregular curvature of the cornea or lens of the eye, resulting in blurring of vision at some angles.

Blinking: An unconscious behavior that massages and bathes the eye, relieves tension around it, and breaks up the habit of staring. Most people with poor eyesight have lost the ability to blink effortlessly and frequently; thus, it is an important vision improvement exercise.

Ciliary muscles: Muscles within the eye, governed by the autonomic nervous system, that release the lens from the tendinous sling that holds it in an oblong shape. This allows the lens to assume a rounder shape, which focuses the eye for near vision.

Fovea centralis: The area of greatest visual acuity within the eye. The fovea is a tiny, pit-shaped area of the retina, at the center of the macula, which contains only cone cells. The nerve cells that overlie the rods and cones in every other part of the retina are pulled aside in this area.

Glaucoma: A condition of excessive fluid pressure within the eye, causing damage (such as nerve fiber destruction and compression of blood vessels), and leading to deteriorating vision or blindness.

Hypermetropia: See *hyperopia.*

Hyperopia: A refractive error, often called *farsightedness,* in which the focal length of the eye is too short. Images are focused behind the retina rather than on it, rendering near vision inadequate.

Macula: Full name *macula lutea,* the area at the center of the retina where detailed vision is possible. Vision is sharpest at the center of the macula, called the *fovea.*

Macular degeneration: Central blindness resulting from death of the macula cells, preventable with eye exercises.

Myopia: A refractive error, also called *nearsightedness,* in which the focal length of the eye is too long. Images are focused in front of the retina rather than on it, rendering distant vision inadequate.

Palming: A vision improvement exercise believed by vision improvement teachers to rest the optic nerve and the muscles within and around the eye, relax the nervous system, and amplify the effect of other eye exercises. Palming is usually done in a darkened room, with the hands lightly covering the eye orbits, touching the cheekbones and forehead while blackness or darkness is envisioned.

Presbiopia: A condition in which the lens hardens, and then does not become convex enough for the eye to see well in the near field. This is know as "forty's farsightedness."

Reiki: From the Japanese phrase meaning "universal life force," a form of touch therapy in which energy is conducted from one person to another through a gentle laying on of hands.

Retina: A network of nerve cells in the rear of the eye, which translates light rays into neural information.

Retinoscope: An instrument for measuring the direction and extent of refractive errors.

Saccadic movements: The eye's normal small, jerky movements as it moves its fixation from one small point to another. Saccadic movements are too rapid to be visible.

Shifting: An exercise used by vision improvement teachers to create fluidity and flexibility in the gaze by imitating the anatomically appropriate use of the eyes, in which they move effortlessly from one small detail to another.

Skying: A variant of the sunning vision improvement exercise for cloudy, overcast days. Skying is done with open eyes, looking away from the sun, with a smaller rotation of the head than in sunning.

Soft eyes: The opposite of the "frozen stare" that is the hallmark of bad eyesight, and characteristic of good eyesight and healthy eyes. A soft gaze moves easily from one small detail to another, accepting what it sees.

Sternocleidomastoids: A pair of neck muscles, originating from the breastbone and clavicle and inserting into the mastoid (a small, bony projection below the ear). These muscles work together to bend the head forward. Either of them, working alone, rotates the head to the opposite side or bends it toward the shoulder of the same side.

Sunning: A vision improvement exercise designed to teach the eyes to adjust to a wide range of intensities of light. Sunning is done in mild sunshine, facing the sun, with the eyes lightly closed, often with self-massage around the eyes, and with the head or upper body continually rotating through 180 degrees.

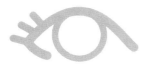

Additional Resources

Bates, William H. *The Bates Method for Better Eyesight without Glasses.* New York: Henry Holt, 1986 (revised edition; paperback).

———. *The Cure of Imperfect Sight by Treatment without Glasses.* CITY: Health Research, 1978.

Huxley, Aldous. *The Art of Seeing.* New York: Harper, 1942

Schneider, Meir. *The Movement for Self Healing.* Novato, California: New World Library, 2004.

For more information on the work of Meir Schneider, or to schedule individual sessions, vision improvement classes, or company trainings to decrease eyestrain in front of computers and increase the health of the eye and body for better performance in the workplace, please contact:

The School for Self-Healing
2218 48th Avenue
San Francisco, CA 94116-1551
Ph: (415) 665-9574. Fax: (415) 665-1318.
www.self-healing.org
email: info@self-healing.org